Contents

BPP
UNIVERSITY
SCHOOL OF HEALTH

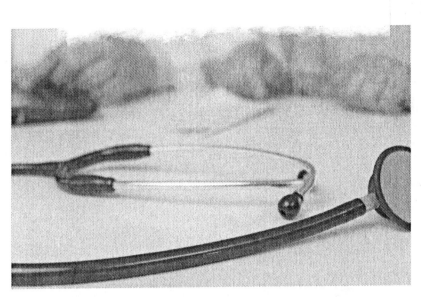

Succeeding in the MRCGP CSA

Common scenarios and revision notes for the Clinical Skills Assessment

Second Edition

Milan Mehta, Chirag Mehta, Khizzer Majid & Lisa Broom

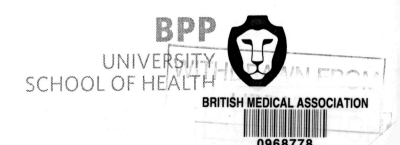

BPP
UNIVERSITY
SCHOOL OF HEALTH

First edition October 2011
Second edition April 2017

ISBN 9781 5097 0764 5
Previous ISBN 9781 4453 7953 1
e-ISBN 9781 5097 0768 3
e-ISBN 9781 5097 0772 0

British Library Cataloguing-in-Publication Data
A catalogue record for this book is available from the British Library

Published by
BPP Learning Media Ltd
BPP House, Aldine Place
London W12 8AA

www.bpp.com/health

Printed in the United Kingdom by
RICOH UK Limited
Unit 2
Wells Place
Merstham
RH1 3LG

Your learning materials, published by BPP Learning Media Ltd, are printed on paper sourced from sustainable, managed forests.

ii

BPP
UNIVERSITY
SCHOOL OF HEALTH

About the Publisher

The UK's only university solely dedicated to business and the professions.

We are dedicated to preparing you for a professional career. We offer a strong commercial approach, within a business culture designed to help you stand out in the workplace after you graduate. Our programmes are designed in partnership with employers and respected professionals in the fields of law, business, finance and health.

Every effort has been made to ensure the accuracy of the material contained within this guide. However it must be noted that medical treatments, drug dosages/formulations, equipment, procedures and best practice are currently evolving within the field of medicine.

Readers are therefore advised always to check the most up-to-date information relating to:

- The applicable drug manufacturer's product information and data sheets relating to recommended dose/formulation, administration and contraindications.
- The latest applicable local and national guidelines.
- The latest applicable local and national codes of conduct and safety protocols.

It is the responsibility of the practitioner, based on their own knowledge and expertise, to diagnose, treat and ensure the safety and best interests of the patient are maintained.

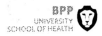

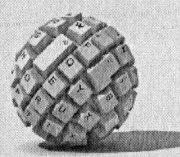

Free Companion Material

Readers can access a blank mark sheet, to use as part of the practice scenarios, for free online.

To access the above companion material please visit **www.bpp.com/freehealthresources**

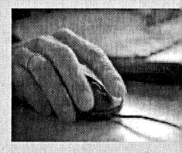

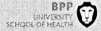

About the Authors

Milan Mehta

Milan Mehta is a GP Partner in the West Midlands, successfully obtaining his MRCGP qualification in 2009. He has published articles in a number of international medical journals and is co-author of the book *Succeeding in the MRCGP AKT*. He enjoys supervising medical students at his practice and he is also a GP trainer. He has also worked as an academic GP at Keele University School of Medicine, where he obtained a Diploma in Medical Education.

Chirag Mehta

Chirag Mehta is a Training Programme Director, GP Trainer and a salaried GP in the West Midlands. He completed the MRCGP in 2011. He is lead author for the book *Succeeding in the MRCGP AKT* and also co-author for a book for medical students on core clinical cases. He has publications in the *BMJ*, the *Public Health* journal and also the RCGP journal for GP trainees, *InnovAiT*. He has a keen interest in medical education and has successfully obtained the Diploma in Medical Education at Keele University.

Khizzer Majid

Khizzer Majid is a GP Principal in the West Midlands. Having successfully completed the MRCGP in 2010, he is able to pass on relevant and up-to-date experience of the CSA examination. Alongside general practice, he is currently involved with improving GP ST3 training.

Lisa Broom

Lisa Broom is a GP in the West Midlands. She divides her work between a salaried role and locum sessions, giving her the opportunity to experience different healthcare systems and practices. She completed her MRCGP in 2016, having taken her CSA exam at the new RCGP headquarters, and achieved an award in recognition of her high score in the AKT examination in 2015.

BPP
UNIVERSITY
SCHOOL OF HEALTH

Acknowledgements

We would like to thank all our friends and family who have wholeheartedly supported us during the writing of this book.

Special thanks to Sarah Gear who kindly agreed to peer review the original edition of this book for us. She is a lady with bundles of positive energy that made her an excellent mentor during our GP vocational training and she has inspired us to contribute something to teaching and learning in the medical profession. Her constructive suggestions and comments (which often made us smile!) have undoubtedly made this title a much stronger revision aid.

We would also like to thank Abhijit Bhattacharyya and Rodger Charlton for their helpful thoughts and feedback.

Finally, we would like to thank Lisa Broom for joining our team of authors and particularly for writing the new CSA circuit for this edition.

Abbreviations

A&E	Accident & Emergency unit
ACE	angiotensin converting enzyme
ACR	albumin:creatinine ratio
AF	atrial fibrillation
AKT	applied knowledge test
ALT	alanine transaminase
AUDIT	alcohol use disorders identification test
bd	twice daily
BASH	British Association for the Study of Headache
BMI	body mass index
BP	blood pressure
BPH	benign prostatic hyperplasia
BTS	British Thoracic Society
CHC	combined hormonal contraception
CKD	chronic kidney disease
COPD	chronic obstructive pulmonary disease
CN	cranial nerves
CRP	C-reactive protein
CSA	clinical skills assessment
CT	computerised tomography
CVD	cardiovascular disease
DIPJ	distal interphalangeal joint
DNA	did not attend
DPP4	dipeptidyl peptidase 4
DVT	deep vein thrombosis
DVLA	Driver and Vehicle Licensing Authority
eGFR	estimated glomerular filtration rate
EC	emergency contraception
ECG	electrocardiogram
EEG	electroencephalogram
ENT	ear, nose and throat
ESR	erythrocyte sedimentation rate
FBC	full blood count
FH	family history
GAD	generalised anxiety disorder
GCA	giant cell arteritis

GGT	gamma-glutamyl transpeptidase
GI	gastrointestinal
GLP-1	glucagon-like peptide 1
GP	general practitioner
GTN	glyceryl trinitrate
GU	genito-urinary
GUM	genito-urinary medicine
HAD	hospital anxiety and depression scale
HIV	human immunodeficiency virus
HRT	hormone replacement therapy
INR	international normalised ratio
IPSS	International Prostate Symptom Score
IUD	intrauterine device
IV	intravenous
IVDU	intravenous drug user
LFT	liver function tests
LUTS	lower urinary tract symptoms
LMP	last menstrual period
MCPJ	metacarpophalangeal joint
MCV	mean corpuscular volume
MRCGP	Membership of the Royal College of General Practitioners
MIDAS	migraine disability assessment score
MRI	magnetic resonance imaging
od	once daily
NICE	National Institute for Health and Clinical Excellence
nocte	at night
NOAC	new oral anticoagulant
NSAID	non-steroidal anti-inflammatory drug
OA	osteoarthritis
OTC	over-the-counter
PE	pulmonary embolism
PEFR	peak expiratory flow rate
PHQ-9	patient health questionnaire
PIL	patient information leaflet
PIPJ	proximal interphalangeal joint
PMH	past medical history
PMR	polymyalgia rheumatica
PO	per os (to be taken orally)

POP	progestogen-only pill
PPI	proton pump inhibitor
PR	per rectum
prn	as required
PSA	prostate specific antigen
PV	per vaginum
qds	four times daily
RCGP	Royal College of General Practitioners
RR	respiratory rate
SGLT-2	sodium/glucose cotransporter 2
SIGN	Scottish Intercollegiate Guidance Network
SOB	shortness of breath
SSRI	selective serotonin reuptake inhibitor
STD	sexually transmitted disease
STI	sexually transmitted infection
TIA	transient ischaemic attack
tds	three times daily
TFT	thyroid function tests
TURP	transurethral resection of prostate
U&E	urea and electrolytes
UPSI	unprotected sexual intercourse
UTI	urinary tract infection

Foreword

It is a pleasure to write a foreword for the second edition of this very successful book. Since the first edition was published in 2011 we have learnt a bit more about what it takes to pass the MRCGP Clinical Skills Assessment, a complex and, for some, frustrating assessment.

In some ways it's easy: treat each new case as a new patient in your own surgery, listen closely to what they are saying and respond to the unique story they are telling you. But we know it is never that straightforward. Countless trainees have struggled to pass, whilst getting excellent feedback in their practices from patients and trainers alike. So what is the trick? Well, there are several things not to do: don't work your way through a formulaic checklist as though you are trying to get a car though its MOT, don't ask questions then not listen or respond to the answers and don't use jargon – not just medical terms like 'I see you had a Non-STEMI in the past' but also 'what are your expectations'. There are also positive things you can do: look and sound like you care about this patient and their story, use all the types of language at your disposal to build a relationship, fleeting and of-the-moment as it will be. Maybe (cautiously) have a joke if it seems appropriate, use and respond to small talk to create a partnership with the patient, to reassure them (and the examiner) that you know what you are doing. Pay attention, work fast and have a plan. Most people who fail struggle with time management, taking too long in the first third of the consultation to get to a satisfactory closure.

The authors of this book have called on the collective experience of their own success in this exam and their expertise as trainers. They know that the route to success is through practice. The cases they have developed allow you to practise with friends and colleagues, so you can gain the confidence you need to give succinct and easily understood explanations. Please do take the opportunity to video yourself as you work with these cases in groups, so you can watch yourself and develop insight into your strengths and weaknesses.

I wish you every success.

Kay Mohanna
Professor of Values Based Healthcare Education
Worcester University Institute of Health and Society

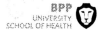

Preface to second edition

This new revised edition is the result of updating the original cases, but now also providing you with an entire new circuit of CSA cases to work through, based on the latest evidence-based guidance.

The original edition received so much positive feedback (which was an absolute delight!), so this new edition has been written with the original format in mind. However, this book includes new cases to increase the range of clinical topics covered, but the cases have also been written to be even more diverse to reflect the patients we see in real-life General Practice.

The chapters 'About the CSA' and 'Useful advice for the CSA' have been updated to reflect the fact that the CSA exam is now held at the RCGP headquarters in Euston, London.

As with the original edition, use this book to help give you a structured, sensible approach to apply to any case you may encounter in the CSA exam, but also in your day-to-day clinics. Remember, the earlier you start using this book, the more benefits you will gain from it!

We wish you the best of luck with the CSA exam and in your careers as GPs of the future!

Milan Mehta, Chirag Mehta, Khizzer Majid & Lisa Broom
January 2017

Preface to first edition

This book will hopefully be a useful aid to helping you overcome one of the biggest hurdles in obtaining your MRCGP which you will need in order to qualify as a GP. Whilst this book will mostly be applicable to GP ST3s, it will still be valuable to GP trainees at any stage in their training.

It is important to realise from the beginning that there is no one single book that can be solely used to pass the CSA exam. As you will have heard many times before, you will learn much more from your patients than you will from any textbook. Therefore, the best exam practice you will ever get is by seeing plenty of patients in your own clinics, learning from the wide variety of problems that they present with and by reflecting on how your consultations went. Passing the CSA will mean that you can communicate effectively with patients, understand their problems, address their concerns and produce mutually agreed management plans.

Whilst this book could never promise to teach you everything about every medical condition, the main strength of this book lies in the fact that it will help give you a structured, generalised approach that you can apply to any case that you may see in clinic or, indeed, in the CSA exam! In addition, you will also have two CSA circuits worth of cases to role-play and to think about how you would tackle them. There are also helpful suggestions under each of the domains you will be assessed on for each case along with useful phrases to help you explore and discuss difficult issues with patients.

Remember, the earlier you use this book in preparation for your CSA exam, the more benefits you will reap from it.

We wish you the best of luck!

Milan Mehta, Chirag Mehta & Khizzer Majid
October 2011

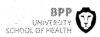

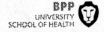

The Clinical Skills Assessment (CSA) and how to use this book

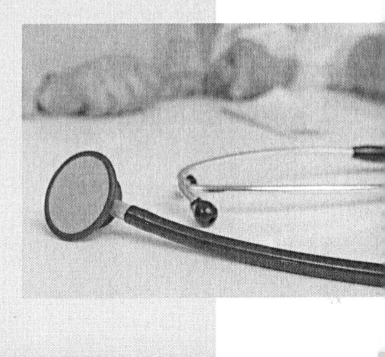

About the CSA

The Clinical Skills Assessment is now an essential part of the MRCGP. The Royal College of General Practitioners says it is 'An assessment of a doctor's ability to integrate and apply appropriate clinical, professional, communication and practical skills in general practice'.

When and where does the CSA take place?

The CSA is held at least seven times a year at RCGP headquarters at 30 Euston Square, London NW1.

How to apply to do the CSA

It is only eligible to GP ST3s and they have to apply online for this. The information regarding dates and application are on the RCGP website (www.rcgp.org.uk/training-exams/mrcgp-exams-overview/mrcgp-exam-applications.aspx).

Format of the CSA

The exam lasts three hours and each candidate is allocated a consulting room and has 13 patients. Each consultation will last a maximum of 10 minutes and may involve a patient coming into your room or it may involve you going to another room for a home visit scenario or a telephone consultation. All patients are played by skilled simulated patients who perform their role in a consistent manner and each consultation has its own examiner who marks the same case all day in order to maintain calibration. An examiner will accompany each patient into your consulting room but they will not play a part in the consultation (except to hand you information at certain points) and you should essentially ignore the examiners.

The exam will contain one paediatric case (it may be a parent presenting with concerns about their child, or occasionally a child may be present).

How is the CSA marked?

The cases assess different aspects of the RCGP curriculum and are designed to reflect the diversity and range of patients and their problems that are seen in general practice. The examiner marks each consultation according to three domains – data gathering, clinical management and interpersonal skills.

Data-gathering, technical and assessment skills

- Gathering and using data for clinical judgement, choice of examination, investigations and their interpretation

- Demonstrating proficiency in performing physical examinations and using diagnostic and therapeutic instruments

Clinical management skills

- Recognition and management of common medical conditions in primary care

- Demonstrating a structured and flexible approach to decision-making

- Demonstrating the ability to deal with multiple complaints and co-morbidity

- Demonstrating the ability to promote a positive approach to health

Interpersonal skills

- Demonstrating the use of recognised communication techniques to gain understanding of the patient's illness experience and develop a shared approach to managing problems

- Practising ethically with respect for equality and diversity issues, in line with the accepted codes of professional conduct

Each of these domains carries the same number of marks. The marks from all three domains are then added together to create a final mark for each consultation. The pass mark for the exam is created using the borderline group method. This means that as

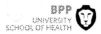

well as you receiving a mark for the sum of the three domains for each consultation, the examiner will also give you an overall comment of pass, fail or borderline. For each consultation the borderline marks are added and then averaged. This process is done for all the 13 consultations and the average borderline score for each is totalled. This creates the cut score which is then adjusted to make the final pass mark taking into account the standard error of measurement.

Exam day

On the day itself, make sure you bring valid photo identification – ie passport or photo driving licence, as nothing else will be accepted. You also need to bring your doctor's bag and certain equipment which you will find listed in the document entitled 'CSA Information For Candidates' which you can find on the RCGP web link above. This document will also provide you with important general information about the CSA exam. On the day of the exam, you will be asked to transfer your equipment into a clear plastic bag which will provided. Any other equipment required will be given to you in the room. On your desk, there will be a list of all the patients you will see in your surgery along with some background information. There will also be some blank FP10 prescriptions and 'fit notes' and some notepaper for you to scribble on.

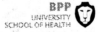

Useful advice for the CSA

Our own experience of the CSA

We all remember turning up for our CSA exam, whether it was at the old centre in Croydon, or the new RCGP headquarters in Euston Square. The new RCGP headquarters has a separate examinations entrance where all candidates initially gather in the lobby area before being ushered upstairs to the examination floors. The area for the examination was surprisingly welcoming, with a tea and coffee area to relax in during the break in the middle of the exam. The 'consulting rooms' are much larger than you might imagine, and all have views of either the road or the internal courtyard.

The exam was three hours long but at least we had our own consulting rooms and were not expected to move rooms for the cases. As soon as the initial buzzer went and the first patient and examiner walked in, those three hours seemed to fly by very quickly...

It would be a lie to say that, on the day of the exam, the CSA did not feel like the biggest exam we had ever taken in our lives. However, there were certain factors that reassured us and made us go into that exam and perform at our best. These factors included the fact that the exam seemed to be a fair one and that all of the cases we had were common problems that any jobbing GP would be expected to deal with. However, the roles the simulated patients played and their backgrounds were quite varied which is just how they would be in real life. The level of factual knowledge required in each station did not seem too great (as this is already formally assessed in your AKT exam) and so the skills that were being tested in the CSA seemed very different. Speaking clearly and using terms that patients can understand, building up a rapport with them and deciding together how their problems were going to be tackled seemed to be the order of the day.

It did seem slightly strange at the beginning of each station when an examiner would walk into the room virtually hidden behind each patient and would not say very much. However, we soon got used to this after the first couple of patients.

In some stations, it often seemed that we had run out of time before we felt the case had drawn to a proper close, but we at least tried to ensure we had safety-netted every patient appropriately.

Leading up to the exam

It may seem a bit clichéd, but it is really important to think of every patient during your time in general practice as being a potential learning opportunity. Whether you see a patient with heart failure or eczema, always make a note of any questions that spring to mind (eg what different treatment options are available? Are there national guidelines on this topic? Did I have the relevant knowledge to answer their questions?). You can then use these learning objectives you generate to help you maximise the learning potential from all your patients.

It will also be useful to imagine each patient you see as if it is your CSA exam. Practising your consultation techniques and structure in your CSA exam that you are going to be using in your everyday surgeries not only will mean that you are constantly preparing for the exam but also you will probably find that both you and your patients will have a better consultation experience. This may be hard to believe initially, but by finding out what is really behind Mrs Jones's repeated attendances, for example, will mean that both you and the patient will end the consultation feeling more satisfied.

Many trainees also use a timer on their desk (that the patients can't see!) so they can practise time management, which is an area many candidates struggle with.

Just before the exam, it would be strongly advisable to stay in a hotel that is as close to the CSA exam centre as possible. You will have enough to worry about on the day itself, without being needlessly stressed by a delayed train, heavy motorway traffic or a punctured tyre on the morning of the exam. There are plenty of hotels (of varying prices) that are all within walking distance of RCGP headquarters.

Tips for the big day itself

Assuming you have had a restful sleep the night before the exam, make sure you wake up in plenty of time to have a good breakfast! You will need the energy to keep you going through the day as you may not necessarily have enough time to eat another proper meal until after the exam has finished.

Once you are told to go to your consulting room, you will have a few minutes to yourself before the actual exam starts. There will be a folder on your desk containing the 'Instructions To Candidates' sections for each case of the exam. Some candidates prefer to quickly glance through these before the exam in order to get those mental cogwheels turning and subconsciously work out what may possibly come up in that case and how they could tackle it. However, other candidates may find looking through folder confuses them even more and so it essentially comes down to personal preference.

Each case will last ten minutes and you will not be required to document the consultation on a computer or on paper. You will then have two minutes between each case to prepare for the next one.

If you want to prescribe anything on a FP10 form or write down any required investigations on request cards (eg blood tests, X-rays), please be aware that anything you write down in the exam will be formally assessed by the examiner during that station. For example, say you wish to prescribe co-amoxiclav 250 mg **tds** for three days for a UTI but you accidentally write down 'co-amoxiclav 250 mg **bd** for 3 days', then this will be marked down by the examiner. An easy way of avoiding this problem is to explain to the patient exactly what you are going to prescribe them and say that you will leave the prescription for them to collect from reception later. This same approach could be used for blood test request forms as long as you explain exactly which tests you are proposing to do eg 'I want to do a blood test to check your thyroid function and your haemoglobin level to see if you are anaemic'. However, the patient may insist they want to have the prescription before they leave the consultation, in which case you know that this is required and that the FP10 you issue will be marked. It is easy to make written mistakes in the heat of the moment and not only can these be avoided, but it may also save you time to explain what you intend to do verbally to the patient and then ask them to collect any forms later on that day (ie so you do not actually need to write them during the CSA station itself!).

Finally, one of the most precious pearls of wisdom to give you is that during the CSA exam, just forget that you are actually in an exam (we know it's easier said than done!). Instead, try your hardest to imagine that you are back in your training practice during one of your usual surgeries. From your own surgeries, you are used to patients walking through your door with almost any problem which you always seem to deal with and manage. Therefore, treat the simulated patients as if they were your own and you will quickly realise that this three-hour surgery is not too dissimilar to the numerous surgeries you have already done so far. Furthermore, you should also feel reassured by the fact you have hundreds of hours of consulting experience which you can call upon during the exam. By embracing this sense of familiarity and using this previous experience, you will have the self-confidence boost you need to overcome any exam nerves!

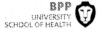

How to get the most out of this book

This book provides you with cases for 3 CSA exam circuits (13 cases per circuit). Each case is accompanied by the instructions that both the exam candidate and simulated patient would be given.

The best thing to do is to go through these cases with friends or peers because by role-playing the cases you will develop a better feel for, and understanding of them. For example, in playing the role of the candidate, you will try to identify the patient's reason for consultation, what is on their agenda and then you will formulate a shared management plan. However, when you then play the role of that patient, you will be able to clearly see what the patient's agenda was and can then work out, retrospectively, what other questions you could have asked in order to elicit that information. You could also think about other ways you could have addressed their fears, concerns and expectations.

After role-playing the cases, you should then seek constructive feedback from your revision group in terms of what was done well and what could be done differently. This should cover aspects such as:

- Clinical factors – such as points on history and examination.

- Communication skills – are there any different ways you could have phrased things so the patient would have understood you better? Do you speak in a soft, friendly tone?

- Non-verbal factors – do you appear attentive enough? Do you make enough eye contact? Do you have any mannerisms which may be slightly off-putting to the patient that you can consciously control?

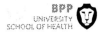

Once you have considered and addressed these points of feedback from your peers you should then read the accompanying notes that are given with each case. These notes will give specific advice under each of the domains that the cases are marked on:

- Data gathering, technical and assessment skills
    - Advice on specific points of history and examination
    - Any red flag symptoms you should not miss

- Interpersonal skills
    - Advice on how to elicit the patient's ideas, concerns and expectations

- Clinical management
    - Treatment options available with advice on areas of discussion to have with the patient about them

    - Advice on how to safety net to ensure patients are appropriately followed up

At the end of the cases, you will also be given useful suggestions for further reading in case you wish to enhance your clinical knowledge and/or answer any further learning objectives you may have come up with.

By going through this process of role-playing, giving each other feedback and then completing any further learning objectives you create, you will rapidly see your consultation skills improve.

It is also extremely useful to discuss different ways in which all members of your revision group would have approached the same cases. As you will already know, there is never only one correct way to do a consultation. Therefore, by discussing different approaches you will gradually obtain and develop your own armoury of consultation skills.

The cases in this book will serve as a guide on how to approach the cases in the exam, but you can take this learning even one step further by creating new cases with your peers. By sitting down and thinking about what will happen in each case and what both the doctor and patient will want from the consultation, you are already (and maybe unknowingly) pushing yourself to use your consultation skills at a much higher level, which can only result in a better performance on the day itself!

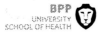

How to approach the cases

The cases are all marked according to the same three domains of data gathering, clinical management skills and interpersonal skills. For any case, here are some general aspects that you should try to include which will improve your consultation skills and, as a consequence, will also help you maximise your score.

Start the consultation by introducing yourself and using an open-ended question such as 'Hello, my name is Dr X. What's brought you in to see me today?'

Give patients ample time at the start to speak without interruption and listen carefully whilst encouraging them to give you the information you require. Examples of this active listening include nodding your head and also the use of verbal gestures such as 'Hmm ... I see.' Also, maintaining good eye contact with the patient is important.

It is important to respond to both verbal and non-verbal cues by the patient and explore these in more depth. A verbal cue may include a patient saying to you that a close relative or friend has recently passed away. Be sure you acknowledge this by saying something like 'I'm really sorry to hear that.' It is easy to get overwhelmed with time pressure during the exam and a common pitfall is to not listen properly to what your patients are saying to you. This will reduce your score in the 'Interpersonal Skills' domain for that station and will possibly prevent your patient from giving you important information if they feel that you have been insensitive by not listening to important things they have just told you. Non-verbal cues may include a patient appearing upset but not having mentioned why. You should acknowledge by saying a phrase such as 'You seem upset – would you like to talk about this?'

The data you gather should include how the problem has affected the patient as a whole and in every important aspect of their life. Ask them how their problem has affected their activities of daily living, their home life, their families, their work and other social activities (eg hobbies, meeting people).

You must always explore the patient's ideas, concerns and expectations. Here are three possible questions you could ask the patient to elicit these thoughts and beliefs:

- 'So what do you think has caused this problem?' – elicits their ideas

- 'Is there anything that is worrying you?'– elicits their concerns

- 'Was there anything in particular you were hoping I could do for you today?' – elicits their expectations

Your data gathering needs to be detailed enough to allow you to both exclude any 'red flag' symptoms and also to arrive at an appropriate diagnosis. This is achieved by asking both open and closed questions. It is important to make sure you ask about all the cardinal symptoms for whichever body system the problem is related to. For example, in a patient with shortness of breath, you would need to ask about both cardiac and respiratory symptoms. Finally, also make sure you specifically ask about red flag symptoms – eg in a smoker with a persistent productive cough, you would ask about weight loss, anorexia, haemoptysis, etc.

Even though it will not be required for every case during the exam, you need to be able to perform an adequate mental or physical examination that is appropriate for the case you are doing. This would be no different to seeing a real patient with the same problem presenting to you in your surgeries as a GP ST3.

In terms of making your consultation most effective, it is vital that you check your patient has understood everything you have said and vice versa and be sure to leave some time for both of you to ask questions at the end. Once you have established a diagnosis, explain this clearly to the patient in language they

 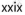

understand whilst using simple terms and avoid medical jargon as much as possible. This may even involve using diagrams to help patients understand difficult concepts and provide them with patient information leaflets which are always a valuable source of information.

The next step is to then explain to patients what all of the available management options are and then, after some discussion, both of you should reach a mutually agreed management plan. There will not always be a single, correct answer but the important thing is to keep the consultation patient-centred and to reach a shared management plan by discussion and negotiation with the patient.

Finally, once you have ensured the patient understands the plan, always remember to include appropriate safety-netting and inform them if they have to be followed-up. Safety-netting involves giving patients advice on what to do if they develop red flag symptoms eg 'Call 999 if your chest pain does not go away within 15 minutes of using your GTN spray.' Follow-up of a problem will vary greatly depending on factors such as whether it is acute or chronic. You should specify whether they should see a GP again after a fixed interval (eg after two to three days or in one month) or to re-present if the problem returns. However, if you are not asking them to come back after a fixed time interval, always remember to give them clear advice on when (and under what circumstances) they should see their GP again.

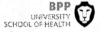

CSA Circuit 1

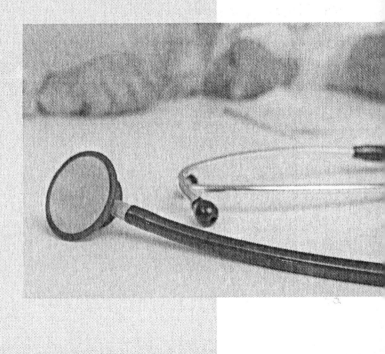

1. Breast cancer screening

Instructions to candidates

Name: Joanne Eardley
Age: 42 years old

Instructions to patients

Opening statement

I've got a history of breast cancer in my family and it has got me a bit worried.

Background

- You are Joanne Eardley, a 42-year-old dental hygienist.

- You divorced 6 months ago and have 3 children (aged 9, 13 and 15 years old).

- You are seeing the GP today as one month ago, your dad's sister died from breast cancer aged 63 years old.

- This aunt was diagnosed with breast cancer a year ago, but was told by doctors that it was 'too advanced to be treated'.

- You were very close to her and her death has caused you a great deal of concern over the possibility of developing breast cancer yourself. No one else in your family (male or female) has any form of cancer.

- No one in your family is known to carry the 'breast cancer genes'.

- You regularly self-examine your breasts and have not found any lumps or anything that concerns you.

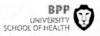
BPP
UNIVERSITY
SCHOOL OF HEALTH

- You are looking for reassurance from the GP that you are not at high risk of breast cancer due to your family history of it.

- You breastfed all your children until up to 6 months to 1 year.

- Your periods are regular (every 28 days) and you had your first period aged 12 years old.

- You have never used any form of hormonal contraception since you are known to get severe migraines during which your speech becomes slurred.

- You have no other medical problems. You have no known drug allergies.

- You are a British Caucasian.

Data gathering, technical and assessment skills

History

- Does she have any history of breast problems/cancers herself?

- Any family history of breast cancer:

  - First degree relatives – mother, father, children, siblings

  - Second degree relatives – grandparents, grandchildren, aunts, uncles, half sister, half brother

  - Third degree relatives – great grandparent, great grandchild, great uncle, great aunt, first cousin, grand nephew, grand niece

  - Paternal history: ≥ 2 relatives diagnosed with breast cancer on father's side of family

- Any family history of unusual cancers?

  - Bilateral breast cancer
  - Male breast cancer
  - Ovarian cancer

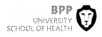

1. Breast cancer screening

- Sarcoma at age < 45 years old
- Glioma or childhood adrenal cortical carcinoma
- Complicated patterns of multiple cancers at young age

- Contraceptive history and/or use of HRT:

  - Slightly high risk if taken long-term, but this decreases when they are stopped

  - Risk from HRT only begins after five years of use

- Obstetric/gynaecology history:

  - Early menarche (aged < 11 years old)

  - Late menopause (aged > 55 years old)

  - Number of children: more children = reduced risk of breast cancer

- Other: raised alcohol intake; diet high in saturated fats

Red flags
Does she have any symptoms of breast cancer?
- Lumps in breasts or under arms
- Nipple retraction or inversion
- Blood-stained nipple discharge
- Breast pain (but cancerous lumps are often painless)
- Changes in skin of breasts (eg peau d'orange)

Examination
- Breast examination only required if patient has any symptoms of breast disease themselves (always offer a chaperone to be present)

BPP
UNIVERSITY
SCHOOL OF HEALTH

Interpersonal skills

Ideas, concerns, expectations

- You need to explore her reasons that she has come to see you today. Does she have breast symptoms herself that she is worried about? Has something happened to someone in her family recently that has triggered her to see you?

- Acknowledge the fact you have heard her saying her aunt has recently died from breast cancer and be empathic about this.

- Try to identify what it is exactly that she wants you to provide for her (eg reassurance, referral for genetic counselling).

Clinical management

- Reassure her that according to NICE guidance, she has < 3% chance of developing breast cancer (as she only had one relative with breast cancer aged > 40 years old, no family history of unusual cancers or Jewish ancestry and no paternal family history).

- Offer referral to local genetics service so they can give her more in-depth advice on her risk of developing breast cancer.

- Advise her that she will have 3-yearly breast screening from the age of 50 as there would be no reason to increase her radiation exposure by starting the screening any earlier.

- Give her verbal or written information on:
  - Breast awareness
  - Lifestyle advice (eg on HRT/oral contraceptives, diet, alcohol, breastfeeding, family size)
  - Contact details of local and national support groups

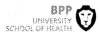

Safety net

- If any red flag symptoms then advise her to come back and see you straight away.

- Advise her to see you again if her family history changes, as this will obviously affect her risk of developing breast cancer too.

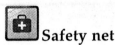

Further reading

NICE (2015) *Familial breast cancer: classification, care and managing breast cancer and related risks in people with a family history of breast cancer.* [Online]. Available at:
www.nice.org.uk/Guidance/CG164
[Accessed 28 February 2017].

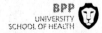

2. Confidentiality and mental capacity

Instructions to candidates

Name:	Ethel Higginbottom
Age:	82 years old
Past medical history:	Angina
	Hypertension
Current medications:	Aspirin 75 mg od
	Atenolol 50 mg od
	Amlodipine 5 mg od
	Isosorbide mononitrate 10 mg bd
	Ramipril 5 mg od
	Simvastatin 40 mg nocte
	GTN spray 1–2 puffs prn
Social history:	Lives alone in a bungalow

Instructions to patients

Opening statement

Doctor, I'm worried about my mum. I don't think she's taking all her tablets.

Background

- You are Janet Saunders (Ethel's daughter).

- You wanted to speak with your mother's GP privately because you are concerned that for the last few weeks she has not been taking her tablets regularly.

- You want to know what medical problems your mother has and why she needs to take all these tablets and whether forgetting to take these medications will affect her health.

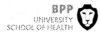

2. Confidentiality and mental capacity

- You do not know which medical problems your mother has and you cannot remember which medications she takes.

- You feel your mother has been suffering from mild memory problems for the last year (eg forgetting birthdays, people's names, paying bills).

- You wonder whether her forgetting to take her medications regularly has affected her memory or if she has dementia.

- Your mother is completely safe at home (eg still always remembers to switch the gas and electric fire off).

- Your mother is fully independent and self-caring. You visit her twice a week at home.

- You wonder if your mother's memory problems can be investigated further.

- You will get frustrated when the doctor initially tells you he cannot give you any of your mother's personal information, but you will then calm down once they explain why they cannot do this and once they reassure you that all of your concerns will be addressed in due course.

Data gathering, technical and assessment skills
History
- Explain from the outset the limitations you are bound by but that you can still listen to Janet's concerns and then take things from there.

- Ask what Janet knows about her mother's medical problems and medications so far.

- Why does Janet think her mother is not taking her medications regularly?

- How long has this problem been going on for?

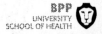

> **Red flags**
> - Does Janet give any information that that suggests her mother may be a danger to herself (eg she forgets to switch the gas off in the kitchen).
> - Any associated neurological symptoms (eg headaches, seizures, focal weakness)?

Interpersonal skills

Ideas, concerns, expectations

- This case is all about exploring the different concerns Janet has about her mum's health.

- You must show that you understand all of Janet's concerns and reassure her that you will address all of them in due course, but whilst also being careful not to divulge Ethel's personal information.

Clinical management

- Ask Janet to state some personal details about her mother (eg Ethel's date of birth, address) to confirm she knows the patient and that you are discussing the correct patient.

- You must inform Janet that you are not allowed to divulge any personal/medical information about her mother, as this would be a breach of patient confidentiality which is deemed to be unethical as stated by the General Medical Council. However, tell Janet you can still listen to her concerns and that you will address these appropriately.

- Explain that the only instance the patient's confidentiality can be breached is if they are a danger to themselves or others. Even then, Janet may not be the person that Ethel's information would have to be divulged to (eg it may be the police or one of your colleagues).

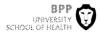

2. Confidentiality and mental capacity

- Explain that you would need to discuss this with Ethel to check that she is okay with her personal/medical information being shared with Janet. But better still, suggest to Janet that she brings her mum along to the next appointment if possible.

- Explain that if Ethel gives consent to her personal/medical information being shared, then Ethel should be advised to book an appointment to see a GP and ask her to bring Janet along then. Ethel's insight into her memory problems could then be assessed with further investigations and possible referral to a memory clinic (with Ethel's consent).

- However, if Ethel chooses not to divulge her personal/medical information with Janet, then this wish would have to be respected by the GP and Janet (as long as Ethel is deemed competent). Even if this happens, reassure Janet that the GP could opportunistically inquire about Ethel's memory problems next time she is seen in clinic or a home visit could be arranged.

Safety net

- Advise Janet that if she feels circumstances change and that Ethel becomes a danger to herself or others, then Janet must inform the GP.

Further reading

1. General Medical Council (2009) *Confidentiality*. [Online]. Available at: www.gmc-uk.org/guidance/ethical_guidance/confidentiality.asp [Accessed 28 February 2017].

2. Department of Health (2003) *Confidentiality: NHS Code of Practice*. [Online]. Available at: www.gov.uk/government/uploads/system/uploads/attachment_data/file/200146/Confidentiality_-_NHS_Code_of_Practice.pdf [Accessed 28 February 2017].

3. HM Government (2005) *Mental Capacity Act 2005*. [Online]. Available at: www.legislation.gov.uk/ukpga/2005/9/contents [Accessed 28 February 2017].

3. Emergency contraception

Instructions to candidates

Name:	Rabia Khan
Age:	19 years old
Past medical history:	None
Social history:	Studying second year of psychology at university

---

Instructions to patients

Opening statement

Hi. I just wondered if I could get the morning-after pill please.

Background

- You are Rabia Khan and you are 19 years old.

- You are in the second year of a psychology degree at university and live away from home. You come from a Muslim family who strictly do not believe in sex before marriage.

- You have been going out with your first-ever boyfriend for the past year (your family are unaware of this). You met him on your course and he is the same age as you.

- Two days ago, you both had unprotected sexual intercourse, which was consensual.

- This was your first ever episode of sexual intercourse with anyone. You have not had any further episodes with anyone since then.

- You want the morning-after pill as you are terrified at the thought of becoming pregnant (as you think your family would disown you, both in terms of contact and also financially).

3. Emergency contraception

- You have not been able to concentrate on your studies at all since this episode.

- You have never used any form of contraception before.

- Your last period was 3 weeks ago and was normal and your cycles are regular (every 28 days).

- Your boyfriend told you he has never had any 'STDs' before.

- You have no medical problems.

- You have never had any pelvic infections before.

- You do not take any medications and you have no drug allergies.

Data gathering, technical and assessment skills

History

- Explore Rabia's reasons for wanting emergency contraception.

- When did she last have unprotected sex? Was it consensual?

- Has she had sex at any other times in the last few days?

- What is their usual method of contraception? Did this method fail and, if so, why (eg missed pills, condom tear)?

- Does she have any contraindications to emergency contraception (eg history of pelvic infections or ectopic pregnancies)?

- Does she have a history of valvular heart disease?

- Is she taking any current medications?

- Is she at risk of STIs – have either of them had any other sexual partners in the last six months?

> **Red flags**
> - STI
> - Could she be pregnant? – always ask about LMP
> - Rape
> - Vulnerable adult

> **Examination**
> - Blood pressure, weight

Interpersonal skills
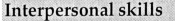

- The key to this case is to show empathy and to build a rapport with her as she is terrified at the prospect of becoming pregnant as she feels that her family would disown her both financially and in terms of communication.

Ideas, concerns, expectations

- 'Why is it so important for you not to be pregnant now?'

- Due to the sensitive nature of this problem (and anxieties regarding her family), reassure her that everything you discuss in this consultation will remain confidential.

- Explore how the morning-after pill and her relationship with her boyfriend are affecting her life in general (eg studies, family).

- Do not let your own personal beliefs affect your consultation with her, as you have a duty as a professional to remain non-judgemental and to be objective. If you do not do this then you will surely lose her trust in you and, therefore, her problem will not have been managed in a just manner.

- Legally, emergency contraception is not the equivalent of procuring a termination.

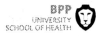

- If you have religious beliefs that prevent you from prescribing the morning-after pill, then you have a duty to help her find another prescriber.

Clinical management

1. Emergency contraceptive pill – either 'Levonelle' or 'ellaOne'

- Levonorgestrel 1.5 mg tablets (Levonelle)
  - Single dose.
  - It is licensed for use up to 72 hours after unprotected sex.
  - Warn patient that the longer the delay in taking this drug, the less effective it will be.
  - Contraindications: acute porphyria.
  - If patient vomits < 2 hours after taking drug, she needs to take another dose (possibly with an anti-emetic).
  - Warn patient she may have some light PV bleeding or spotting and her next period may be delayed by up to a week. If any uncertainty that next period has occurred, do pregnancy test at least three weeks after UPSI.

- Ulipristal Acetate (EllaOne)
  - Single dose; selective progesterone-receptor modulator; efficacy same as Levonelle.
  - It is licensed for use up to 120 hours after unprotected sex.
  - Warn patient that the longer the delay in taking this drug, the less effective it will be.
  - Contraindications: uncontrolled severe asthma, repeated use within a menstrual cycle.

- If patient vomits < 3 hours after taking drug, she will need to take another dose (possibly with an anti-emetic).

- Warn patient she may have some light PV bleeding or spotting and her period may be delayed by up to a week. If any uncertainty that next period has occurred, do pregnancy test at least three weeks after UPSI.

2. Copper IUD

- 'This involves inserting a small copper containing device into the womb.'

- This is the **most effective** method of emergency contraception.

- It is licensed for use up to five days after unprotected sex or five days after ovulation.

- PV swabs need to be taken at the time of IUD insertion (don't forget, this is an 'emergency' procedure).

- Antibiotic cover is needed if at risk of STI.

Safety net

- 'No form of emergency contraception is 100% effective.' Even with emergency contraception, there is still a small possibility she could become pregnant. If this were to happen, she could discuss her options with you at a later date.

- Ask her to do a pregnancy test if next period is abnormally late or if it is very light, heavy or brief and to also see a doctor for review.

- Explain that she will need to use barrier contraception until next period.

- Advise her to see a doctor immediately if develops any lower abdominal pain.

- Despite what her boyfriend has told her, she must be advised that unprotected sex leaves her at risk of STI (including HIV) and that she should ideally get screened for these too at the GUM clinic.

- You must discuss future method of contraception. Even if pregnancy can't be excluded (eg after administering EC), if she remains at risk of pregnancy, you can consider immediately 'quick-starting' CHC, the POP or progestogen-only implant and advising them when to do a pregnancy test.

Further reading

1. Faculty of Sexual and Reproductive Healthcare (2012) *CEU Emergency Contraception Jan 2012.* [Online]. Available at: www.fsrh.org [Accessed 28 February 2017].

2. Faculty of Sexual and Reproductive Healthcare (2009) *CEU Archived Statement Ulipristal (EllaOne) FAQs.* [Online]. Available at: www.fsrh.org [Accessed 28 February 2017].

3. Faculty of Sexual and Reproductive Healthcare (2010) *CEU Quick Starting Contraception.* [Online]. Available at: www.fsrh.org/standards-and-guidance/documents/ ceuguidancequickstartingcontraception/ [Accessed 28 February 2017].

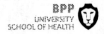

4. Hypertension

Instructions to candidates

Name:	Dennis Hanton
Age:	64 years old
Past medical history:	Hypertension
Current medications:	Bendroflumethiazide 2.5 mg od
	Amlodipine 5 mg od

Instructions to patients

Opening statement

> *I went for my blood pressure check with the nurse. She said it was still high and told me to see you.*

Background

- You are Dennis Hanton, a 64-year-old retired pottery worker.

- You attended your annual blood pressure check with the nurse who advised you to see a doctor as your blood pressure is still a bit high (152/95).

- You have suffered from high blood pressure for the last nine years, but are otherwise well.

- You take bendroflumethiazide 2.5 mg and amlodipine 5 mg once every day.

- Two years ago, another GP previously tried increasing your amlodipine to 10 mg daily, but you could not tolerate the ankle swelling and, therefore, it was reduced back to 5 mg daily and the ankle swelling resolved.

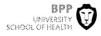

- You then started going to a gym three times per week and improved your diet (less fatty, fried, sweet and salty foods) and your BP fell to within normal limits, until recently however. You also started taking garlic capsules and drinking beetroot juice too.

- You are reluctant to take another drug to control your blood pressure, unless the doctor properly explains to you why you need to take it and what the side effects of the drug are.

- However, you adamantly refuse to have your amlodipine increased again to 10 mg daily due to ankle swelling.

- You have no headaches or visual problems.

- You have no drug allergies.

- You do not drink alcohol and do not smoke.

Data gathering, technical and assessment skills

History

- Does he know why he has to take the tablets and why it is important for his hypertension to be controlled? – check how much he understands.

- Is he taking his tablets regularly – check compliance!

- Has he experienced any side effects from the current medications or any from ones he may have tried in the past?

- What are his views on having to take another medication to control his blood pressure?

- Find out about other cardiovascular risk factors: smoking, dietary habits, level of exercise, etc.

> **Red flags**
> - Recent headaches or visual disturbance? – check to see if he has symptoms of severe hypertension
>
> - (**Note.** 'Accelerated' or 'malignant' hypertension is severe hypertension (systolic BP ≥ 180 mmHg and diastolic BP ≥ 110 mmHg) associated with papilloedema or retinal changes (haemorrhages and exudates).)

Interpersonal skills

Ideas, concerns, expectations

- The key aspects of this case are to check the patient's understanding of the medications that he is taking and to see if he understands why he is taking them.

- It is also important to explore any concerns he may have about taking further medication (eg worries about potential side effects).

Clinical management

- Re-check his BP; pulse; height/weight; waist circumference.

- Before starting an ACE inhibitor, warn patient of their side effects: persistent dry cough, profound light-headedness, renal impairment.

- Check U&E before adding any medication and take opportunity to update CVD risk assessment (eg QRISK2) and use this to help explain why needs another tablet to reduce his cardiovascular risk.

- Start the lowest dose of an ACE inhibitor (eg ramipril 1.25 mg daily).

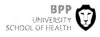

- Ask patient to re-check U&E after seven to ten days (to ensure no renal impairment).

- Re-check BP in four weeks (sooner if any problems) and titrate dose of ramipril upwards accordingly.

Safety net

- Whenever you prescribe an anti-hypertensive drug (or change the dose), always re-check the U&E after seven to ten days to ensure no renal impairment has resulted.

- Advise patient that if he develops any side effects, then he should stop the ramipril and see a doctor as appropriate.

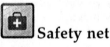

Further reading

1. NICE (2016) *Hypertension in adults: diagnosis and management.* [Online]. Available at: www.nice.org.uk/guidance/cg127 [Accessed 28 February 2017].

2. NICE CKS (2015) *Hypertension – not diabetic.* [Online]. Available at: https://cks.nice.org.uk/hypertension-not-diabetic [Accessed 28 February 2017].

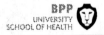

5. Hyperthyroidism

Instructions to candidates

Name: Lisa Foo
Age: 33 years old

Two days ago, Lisa had some blood tests done and the results are shown below:

TSH: 0.10 mU/L   (0.35–5.5 mU/L)
Free T4:   30 pmol/L   (8–22 pmol/L)

Instructions to patients

Opening statement

You wanted to see me again about my thyroid blood test.

Background

- You are Lisa Foo, a 33-year-old pharmacist who is married.

- Your GP asked you to come back to discuss the results of the blood tests you had for your thyroid which you had done earlier this week.

- Your GP requested these blood tests as for the last few weeks you have been losing weight and noticed that your palms are always sweaty and that your hair has become thinner.

- Your periods are usually regular but have recently been longer between bleeds.

- You feel you can no longer tolerate the heat and your hands and fingers keep trembling.

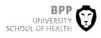

- You have never experienced these problems before.

- There is no one with thyroid problems in your family. However, your younger brother has diabetes and has been injecting insulin since he was a child.

- You have no children yet but are hoping to start a family soon as you fear you may be getting 'too old' to have children.

- You are not on any medications and you have no drug allergies.

Data gathering, technical and assessment skills

History

- Ask about all the symptoms of hyperthyroidism – weight loss, diarrhoea, oligomenorrhoea/amenorrhoea, mood disturbance (irritability, anxiety, psychosis), sweating, palpitations, heat intolerance, tremor, low libido.

- Always ask about both personal and family history of autoimmune problems – eg thyroid problems, Type 1 diabetes mellitus, pernicious anaemia, coeliac disease, vitiligo.

- Drug history – as some drugs can affect thyroid function (especially amiodarone, lithium, thyroxine ingestion).

- It is vital to know if female patients desire to become pregnant soon as this will affect their management options.

Red flags
- Fever > 38.5°C, dehydration, vomiting, seizures, delirium or coma – these are all features of thyrotoxic crisis or storm, which is a medical emergency.

- If they are unwell from any arrhythmias or if there is evidence of cardiac failure, these are medical emergencies too.

Examination

This should have been done in the initial consultation but here is a list for completeness.

- Signs of hyperthyroidism:

  - Hands – sweaty palms, palmar erythema, fine tremor

  - Pulse – tachycardic (is it regular – atrial fibrillation?)

  - Neck – diffuse thyroid enlargement in Graves; multinodular goitre more common in elderly

  - Hair – evidence of thinning or diffuse alopecia

  - Other – brisk reflexes, gynaecomastia, lid lag, urticaria, pruritus, proximal myopathy (muscle weakness +/– muscle wasting)

  - Graves' disease

    - Eyes – exophthalmos, ophthalmoplegia, conjunctival oedema, papilloedema, keratopathy

    - Thyroid acropachy (clubbing)

    - Pretibial myxoedema – swelling above lateral malleoli

    - Diffuse goitre

    - Thyroid bruit

Interpersonal skills

Ideas, concerns, expectations

- You need to find out what her ideas are for what is causing all her symptoms and this should be followed by an explanation of hyperthyroidism using simple terms that she can understand.

- Explain that one of the treatments for hyperthyroidism will mean that she should not conceive during this time – you need to explore whether this will be a realistic treatment option for her.

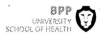

Clinical management

- Beta-blockers – atenolol or propranolol can be used to control symptoms (eg tremors, palpitations) until anti-thyroid therapy becomes effective.

- Refer this lady to Endocrinology to discuss:

  - Carbimazole

    ○ Inhibits thyroid hormone synthesis

    ○ Start carbimazole 10 mg tds

    ○ Risks: agranulocytosis, aplastic anaemia, hepatitis – so need regular FBC/LFT monitoring

  - Radioactive iodine (if carbimazole not effective):

    ○ This takes three to four months to take effect.

    ○ Women of child-bearing age should be advised not to get pregnant for four months.

    ○ Carbimazole should be stopped > 4 days before and re-started > 3 days after this treatment.

    ○ Most will become hypothyroid later (even after many years) after treatment.

    ○ Will need long-term monitoring of TFT after treatment.

Safety net

- Warn patients taking carbimazole that if they get a sore throat (or other infection) that they must stop the drug and see a doctor immediately as they will need an FBC.

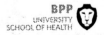

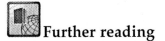

Further reading

1. Kumar P and Clark ML (2009) *Kumar & Clark's Clinical Medicine*. 7th edition. London: WB Saunders.

2. Royal College of Physicians (2007) *Radioiodine in the management of benign thyroid disease. Clinical guidelines: report of a Working Party 2007*. [Online]. Available at: www.thyroiduk.org.uk/tuk/guidelines/Radioiodine%20 guidelines%202007.pdf [Accessed 28 February 2017].

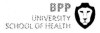

6. Osteoarthritis: home visit

Instructions to candidates

Name: George Cheeseman
Age: 77 years old
Past medical history: Osteoarthritis left hip

Instructions to patients

Opening statement

> *Doctor, I'm in agony with this hip of mine. Can you help me?*

Background

- You are George Cheeseman, a 77-year-old former builder.

- You live alone in a council-owned, terraced house.

- You have asked the GP to visit you at home as your left hip has been much more painful than usual for the last couple of days.

- You have had gradually worsening left hip pain for the last three years.

- A year ago, you had an X-ray of your left hip and the doctor said it showed 'a bit of wear and tear in your hip'.

- Since then you have been taking co-codamol 15/500 tablets which seemed to control the pain until a few weeks ago, after which the pain become progressively worse and has been unbearable for the last two days.

- You saw a physiotherapist for this a year ago, but did not find this helpful.

- You have not fallen or banged your hip against anything.

- The hip pain is normally worst at end of the day and the hip feels stiff – both of these symptoms have become more severe in last two days.

- For the last two days, the pain and stiffness in your hip have limited your mobility so that you have spent most of today in bed due to the pain.

- You feel this is most probably a worsening of the arthritis in your hip and just want something to ease the pain.

- You have no other medical problems. You do not have any drug allergies.

- When asked to be examined, you agree to this, but you are unable to get out of bed due to the pain and wish to be examined whilst lying down in bed.

- You agree to your painkillers being adjusted as suggested by the GP.

- You agree to a see a hip surgeon if the GP explains what different options the hip surgeons may offer to you.

Examination findings of left hip

This is to be given to the candidate after they have performed a hip examination on the patient:

- Left leg is not shortened and is not held in external rotation.

- No redness or swelling around the left hip or groin.

- No tenderness over the left greater trochanter or groin.

- Reduced internal rotation and abduction of the left hip with pain at extremities of movements.

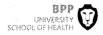

Data gathering, technical and assessment skills

History

- When did this hip pain start? What was the onset (ie sudden or gradual)?

- Is there any associated stiffness/cracking/swelling/redness of the hip?

- Is there any history of trauma/fall to suggest a fracture?

- Are his symptoms related to the time of day?

- What was his former occupation?

- What is he currently taking for pain relief? Is he taking this regularly?

- Does he have any contraindications to NSAIDs?

- Has he previously had physiotherapy? Did it help?

Red flags
- Any fevers/weight loss/sweats or hip pain at night?
- Anything to suggest possible fracture?
- Is the pain constant and unremitting?

Examination
- Can he walk – if so, assess gait (antalgic?).

- If not, examine on bed for any:

  - Obvious leg shortening or is leg held in external rotation (fracture?)

  - Redness/swelling around hip or groin (fracture/bursitis/infection?)

  - Tenderness over greater trochanter or groin (fracture?)

  - Pain at extremes of movement suggest OA (especially if reduced internal rotation and abduction of hip)

BPP
UNIVERSITY
SCHOOL OF HEALTH

Interpersonal skills

Ideas, concerns, expectations

- He is worried that the pain is not going away and wants the pain to be controlled. You will have to explain the likely diagnosis to him and reassure him that pain relief is something straightforward that can be optimised.

Clinical management

This appears to be an acute exacerbation of chronic osteoarthritis of the left hip.

- Reassure patient that there is no evidence of fracture or need for an X-ray (from history or examination) and that it seems most likely to be a severe flare up of his hip OA.

- Check the patient's understanding of osteoarthritis.

- Analgesia:

  - Switch strength of co-codamol to 30/500 tabs (warn of increased risk of constipation, nausea and light-headedness).

  - Consider adding in ibuprofen (max 400 mg tds) and warn to stop NSAID if any abdominal pain/indigestion/ black stools. Do not give NSAID if cardiac disease/renal impairment/asthma/history of GI bleeding.

- Arrange telephone consultation or review 48 hours later to discuss whether needs orthopaedic referral especially if his symptoms are not improving with conservative measures.

- Orthopaedic referral:

  - Hip replacements last 10–15 years, but patient must be warned there is a risk of the hip replacement loosening.

Safety net

  - If pain continues to get worse, then advise them to seek medical attention.

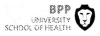

Further reading

1. NICE (2014) *Osteoarthritis: care and management.* [Online]. Available at: www.nice.org.uk/guidance/cg177 [Accessed 28 February 2017].

2. NICE CKS (2015) *Osteoarthritis.* [Online]. Available at: https://cks.nice.org.uk/osteoarthritis [Accessed 28 February 2017].

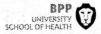

7. Recurrent thrush

Instructions to candidates

Name:	Estelle Smith
Age:	46 years old
Past medical history:	Hypertension
Current medication:	Bendroflumethiazide 2.5 mg od
Social history:	Married; teacher

Instructions to patients

Opening statement

> *Doctor, I keep getting thrush down below and I can't seem to get rid of it.*

Background
- You are Estelle Smith, a 46-year-old teacher and you have been happily married for 22 years.

- You have had several bouts of vaginal thrush over the past 12 months and have now come to see your GP for advice on further treatment.

- One year ago, you had some genital soreness, itching and vaginal discharge (like 'cottage cheese'; not foul smelling), which you thought was thrush and it resolved with Canesten cream from the pharmacy.

- But these symptoms reappeared one month later and you saw another GP who took some vaginal swabs which confirmed it was thrush. He gave you an anti-fungal tablet to take which again cleared the thrush.

- You have had at least five further episodes of thrush which have been treated with 'one-off' tablets or creams.

BPP
UNIVERSITY
SCHOOL OF HEALTH

7. Recurrent thrush

- You have had PV swabs done when your symptoms recurred and these have shown Candida infection on at least two occasions.

- Since your first episode of thrush, your husband has had a few episodes where the end of his penis has been red, sore with some discharge underneath his foreskin. He saw his GP after the first attack who gave him an anti-fungal cream which cleared it up. He has then self-treated with over-the-counter anti-fungal creams after each attack. He told you about this recently as he wondered whether his symptoms were in any way related to your episodes of thrush.

- The thrush has now become a complete nuisance and you feel 'dirty' due to the discharge. It is now starting to affect your sexual relationship with your husband.

- Neither you nor your husband have had other sexual partners during your marriage.

- You have high blood pressure which is well controlled on bendroflumethiazide and are otherwise well.

- You have had no weight loss, lethargy, high thirst or high frequency of urination.

- You are not an IV drug user and have never had a blood transfusion before.

- You have no drug allergies and no family history of medical problems.

Data gathering, technical and assessment skills

History

- Does she have any vulval itching or soreness?

- Is there any vaginal discharge (non-offensive, usually curdy but may be thin)?

- Does it hurt when she has vaginal intercourse (superficial dyspareunia)?

- Does it burn or hurt when she passes urine?

- Contraceptive use:

  - High-oestrogen pill associated with high risk of candidiasis
  - Condom use – because of nonaxyl-9

- Vaginal douching, bubble baths, tight-fitting clothing?

- Definition of recurrent vulvovaginal candidiasis:

  - ≥ 4 documented symptomatic episodes per 12 months

  - Must have moderate/heavy growth of Candida albicans documented on ≥ 2 occasions when symptomatic

---

Red flags
Need to assess for and exclude other causes of recurrent candidiasis:
- Diabetes – check fasting plasma glucose level.

- HIV – multiple sexual partners, IVDU, history of blood transfusions?

- Immunosuppression – are they on chemotherapy or steroids?

Examination
- If 'blind' empirical treatment with topical or tablets fails to work, she will need PV swabs to confirm candidal infection and a PV exam to look for signs of candidiasis or other causes of symptoms.

- Signs of candidiasis: erythema, fissuring, discharge (as above), satellite lesions, excoriation.

Interpersonal skills

Ideas, concerns, expectations

- She is quite distressed that her symptoms have not resolved despite previous treatments. Allow opportunity for the patient to explain how these symptoms have affected her daily life.

BPP
UNIVERSITY
SCHOOL OF HEALTH

- With the recurrent vaginal discharge, she feels 'dirty' and wonders if there is a possibility thrush could be sexually transmitted, even though she does not believe her husband has been unfaithful.

- She is looking for a 'magic cure' to permanently clear her thrush – you will need to educate her on the prognosis of recurrent thrush and treatment options available when you discuss management later.

Clinical management

- Reassure her that thrush is common in women and it does not imply that her husband has been unfaithful! However, in this case it appears that her husband may have developed thrush (candidal balanitis) after Estelle's initial episode and, since they were not both treated at the same time, they may have kept re-infecting each other.

- Since this is the most likely cause of both of their symptoms – offer treatment to Estelle and advise her husband to get anti-fungal treatment from his GP and that they should both treat themselves simultaneously.

- Here are some general management principles for vaginal candidiasis.

General advice

- Avoid perfumed soaps, bubble baths and tight-fitting synthetic clothes.

- Use vulval moisturisers – whilst thrush is not an STI, friction from sexual intercourse may cause tiny tears in the vaginal lining which make it more prone for Candida to thrive and keeping the vagina well moisturised and lubricated may prevent this.

Uncomplicated episode of candidiasis

- Either try topical therapy (eg clotrimazole 500 mg pessary) or oral therapy (fluconazole 150 mg).

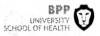

Complicated episode of candidiasis (eg in pregnancy)

- Oral therapy contraindicated, so only treat candidiasis if symptomatic – use any topical antifungal, but for longer seven-day course. No evidence to support treatment of asymptomatic candidiasis.

Recurrent candidiasis

- Try fluconazole 150 mg PO every 72 hours for 3 doses (induction) and then 150 mg once weekly for 6 months (maintenance) and then stop.

- Consider checking FBC, HIV test and fasting glucose to exclude immunosuppression and uncontrolled diabetes/ impaired glucose tolerance as causes.

- Review contraception – recurrent thrush associated with high-oestrogen, so consider low-oestrogen pill or swap to Cerazette or Depo injections (not evidenced, but works in some cases).

- No follow-up needed if symptoms resolve which is what she wants.

- No need to re-test patient after treatment if symptoms have resolved.

- No evidence to treat asymptomatic male sexual partners either in episodic or recurrent vulvovaginal thrush.

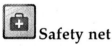Safety net

- If struggling to manage problem in primary care, then refer to GUM clinic for advice on further management and for a full STI screen.

- If recurrent, it is essential to exclude serious underlying causes of recurrent vulvovaginal candidiasis as mentioned above.

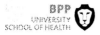

Further reading

British Association of Sexual Health and HIV (2007) *United Kingdom national guideline on the management of vulvovaginal candidiasis.* [Online]. Available at: www.bashhguidelines.org/media/1043/vvc-2007.pdf [Accessed 28 February 2017].

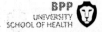

8. Gastroenteritis: telephone consultation

Instructions to candidates

Name:	Kerry Frodsham
Age:	8 years old
Past medical history:	Eczema (well controlled)
Current medication:	None
Social history:	Lives at home with parents

Instructions to patients

Opening statement

Hello doctor. I was wondering if you could visit my daughter today please.

Background

- You are Mr Frodsham (Kerry's father).

- Kerry has diarrhoea and a fever.

- You are requesting a home visit by the doctor as you are worried.

- For the last three days, she has had loose, watery stools (no blood) about three to four episodes times per day.

- She has had no vomiting.

- She is alert and has no obvious abdominal pain.

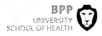

- She is eating less than usual, but still drinking plenty of fluids.

- She is still passing urine normally.

- You have not tried giving her any over the counter medications.

- You cannot see any rash.

- Her hands and feet look pink and feel warm.

- You have no thermometer, but believe she feels a bit warmer than usual.

- Apart from eczema (which is well controlled), she has no other medical problems.

Data gathering, technical and assessment skills
History

- Taking an accurate, clear, focused history is the most important aspect of a telephone consultation, because you do not have the patient sitting in front of you to look at quickly. Plus, you have to be 100% certain you have made an accurate assessment of the patient's state of health over the telephone. If you are at all unhappy with the accuracy of your assessment, you will have to ensure that they are seen by a doctor appropriately (ie either in hospital or at your surgery).

- This is a case of mild gastroenteritis which is most probably viral. Assessing the presence and severity of dehydration is vital. To work this out, you need to ask about inputs (food and fluids – amounts taken) versus outputs (diarrhoea and vomiting – number of episodes per 24 hours), to check she is not at a deficit.

Red flags

- Whilst a viral gastroenteritis is the most likely cause, it is important to remember that diarrhoea can be a part of more serious underlying conditions, which is why it is crucial to ask about red flag symptoms.

- These symptoms include:

  - Photophobia, rash (non-blanching), neck stiffness, headache – meningitis

  - Bloody stools – infective diarrhoea, intussusceptions, colitis

  - Not passing urine or not even drinking small sips of fluids – moderate to severe dehydration

  - Lethargy, drowsiness, floppiness – meningitis or other severe infection/sepsis

- If there is a rash, ask the parents to press a glass over the rash – if the rash is non-blanching, this is **meningococcal septicaemia** until proven otherwise! If this happens, you would call 999 for the patient to go immediately to A&E.

Interpersonal skills

- When parents ring the practice to request a home visit by a doctor, they are often very concerned about the health of their child. They may be very worried about their child's current problem or they are afraid of 'bothering the doctor' and wasting the doctor's time or a combination of these two factors. However, in order to obtain an accurate history, part of your armoury of consultation skills should include the ability to calm a parent/patient down before you can help them.

- The person you speak to on the phone will probably have one or more concerns that need addressing. Whilst you cannot falsely reassure them about everything, by clearly explaining your thought processes, management plan and safety-netting, you will generally have put them more at ease than you realise.

Clinical management

- Explain to Mr Frodshan that you think that this is most likely to be a case of mild gastroenteritis, which is due to a viral infection. Also explain that antibiotics do not work against viruses (since our bodies eliminate viral infections naturally) and that diarrhoea would be a side effect of the antibiotics anyway!

- Advise taking regular paracetamol and if pyrexia is still not controlled, he can add in some ibuprofen (if no history of asthma) and ask him to buy a thermometer if they do not have one.

- Advise plenty of fluids. If Kerry is struggling to take fluids normally, try asking parent to give patient small sips of fluid every 10–15 minutes (this should ensure adequate hydration whilst not overburdening her stomach and causing her to vomit!). Ice lollies are also often a good option.

- Patients usually do not need to be prescribed electrolyte-replacement drinks (eg Dioralyte) if they can tolerate drinking fluids such as fruit juices (since these already contain sufficient electrolytes).

- If there are any red flag symptoms, you will have to decide whether it is most appropriate to call 999 and send the patient urgently to A&E (eg if you suspect meningitis) or for the parents to bring the patient into the surgery to see you immediately.

- If at any point, the patient stops drinking even small sips of fluids to the extent she stops passing urine every 8–12 hours, then she will need to be admitted to hospital to have intravenous fluids and further monitoring.

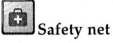
Safety net

- With telephone consultations especially (ie when you cannot see who are you talking to), it is essential establish the details of who you are speaking to (eg name, date of birth, address, relation to patient). If you are not satisfied the person you are speaking to is who they say they are, then you should not divulge any information about the patient to them.

- Make sure you have a much lower threshold for bringing children in to see you in the practice instead of managing them over-the-telephone at home. This is because children have the tendency to deteriorate suddenly and very rapidly!

- Some of these children may still need to see you at the practice as you feel appropriate, based on their clinical need. This is to ensure that their physical state matches the one you assessed earlier in your telephone consultation. When you are having a busy on-call, it is still safer (and sometimes quicker) to take a focused history via telephone and to then just physically examine them when they arrive at your practice later that day. This is so that urgent medical attention can be provided at a much earlier stage than if they were to wait for you to visit them at home or seem them the day after in clinic.

- **Please see a doctor if their symptoms have not improved within 24–48 hours or sooner, if their symptoms have worsened or if you have any concerns.** If you have not admitted the patient, but have brought them in to see you at the surgery, ensure that you have explained the management plan clearly to them, when you want to review them again, red flag symptoms and what to do if they develop any.

- **Please call 111 if you need any medical advice outside your GP surgery's opening hours.**

- As for paediatric cases in general, again, have a low threshold for admission if parents are very worried or concerned. They will know the patient better than anyone and will also know when the patient is not well and these concerns should not be dismissed. This is because doctors often only see a snapshot of the patient's medical problem whereas parents know their child inside out!

Further reading

1. NICE (2009) *Diarrhoea and vomiting in children caused by gastroenteritis in under 5s: diagnosis and management*. [Online]. Available at: www.nice.org.uk/guidance/cg84 [Accessed 28 February 2017].

2. Patient UK (2009) *Acute Diarrhoea in Children*. [Online]. Available at: http://patient.info/health/acute-diarrhoea-in-children [Accessed 28 February 2017].

3. NICE CKS (2013) *Feverish children – management*. [Online]. Available at: https://cks.nice.org.uk/feverish-children-management [Accessed 28 February 2017].

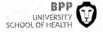

9. Viral labyrinthitis: home visit

Instructions to candidates

Name:	Rajesh Kathirmangamathan
Age:	36 years old
Past medical history:	Nil
Social history:	Lives with flatmate

Instructions to patients

Opening statement

I just feel so dizzy and I can't stop being sick.

Background

- You are Rajesh Kathirmangamathan and are 36 years old.

- You have asked the doctor to visit you at home as you feel so 'dizzy' that you cannot get out of bed.

- A few days ago, you started off with a dry cough, runny nose and sore throat. These symptoms have eased a lot, but are still present.

- For the last 24 hours, you have felt 'dizzy' (ie the room keeps spinning around) and feel unsteady on your feet.

- You have not felt able to leave your bed during this time due to these symptoms.

- You feel your symptoms ease when you remain lying down but worsen when you turn your head or sit up.

- You have also vomited three times today, with no blood in the vomit.

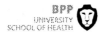

- During this time, you have also felt slightly deaf in both ears.

- There is no discharge from your ears and there is no ringing noise in your ears.

- You do not have any numbness/weakness/pins and needles in your limbs.

- You do not have any rash, neck stiffness or headache.

- You do not have any sensitivity to light or any visual problems.

- You have never had any ear problems before. You have no other medical problems.

- You have no drug allergies.

Data gathering, technical and assessment skills

History

- Clarify what is meant by 'dizzy' – does he mean the room feels like it is spinning around (ie true rotational vertigo) or does he feel light-headed (ie like they are about to faint)? It is important to differentiate between these two, as they both have different causes.

- What were the onset and severity of vertigo like? – sudden, severe onset suggests viral labyrinthitis or even possibly a TIA.

- Is there any associated nausea and vomiting?

- Is there any concurrent hearing loss? – occurs with viral labyrinthitis in affected ear.

- Are there any associated upper respiratory tract infection symptoms (eg runny nose, sore throat, cough) either just before or at the same time as the vertigo? If yes, then it is most likely to be a viral labyrinthitis.

- Other causes of labyrinthitis: TIA/stroke, migraine, subarachnoid haemorrhage, Ménière's disease, vertebrobasillar insufficiency, brain tumour.

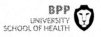

- In benign positional vertigo, there are no interval symptoms between acute attacks (ie they are not dizzy all the time).

- In Ménière's disease, there is also a sense of fullness in the affected ear.

Red flags
- Is there any neck stiffness/photophobia/headache? – may be a subarachnoid haemorrhage or consider meningitis if fever or rash also present.

Examination
- Check vital signs: temperature, pulse, BP, respiratory rate.

- Inspect ears and tympanic membranes with an otoscope.

- Examine cranial nerves – if any nerve apart from CN VIII affected, this is very significant.

- Check hearing with Rinne's and Weber's tests – to exclude a unilateral deafness (but can still happen in labyrinthitis).

- Look for nystagmus – with repetitive testing, nystagmus fades in peripheral vestibular disorders but persists in central lesions.

Interpersonal skills

Ideas, concerns, expectations
- It may be difficult for the patient to talk much depending on how incapacitated he is by his symptoms.

- It is most important to exclude any red flags in the history and find out how severely the symptoms have affected him.

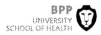

Clinical management

Viral labyrinthitis is usually self-limiting, but may be chronic or recurrent in some people.

- During acute episodes, advise the patient to rest with his eyes closed.

- Warn patient that the nausea, vomiting and vertigo may take a few days to a few weeks to resolve in labyrinthitis.

- Try oral prochlorperazine or cyclizine to ease nausea, vomiting or vertigo. If he is unable to take anything orally, try buccal prochlorperazine.

- If he has sudden onset, unilateral hearing loss, arrange urgent hospital admission in case he has acute ischaemia affecting the brainstem or labyrinth. Emergency treatment may save his sense of hearing.

Safety net

- Advise him to seek medical attention if symptoms worsen (ie double vision, slurred speech, unable to walk properly, focal weakness or numbness).

- Advise him not to drive or operate heavy machinery whilst symptomatic or whilst taking medication, as appropriate.

- If labyrinthitis is chronic or recurrent, arrange ENT referral to exclude sinister pathology.

Further reading

1. NICE CKS (2010) *Vertigo*. [Online]. Available at: https://cks.nice.org.uk/vertigo [Accessed 28 February 2017].

2. Simon C, Everitt H and van Dorp F (2009) *Oxford Handbook of General Practice*. 3rd edition. Oxford: Oxford University Press.

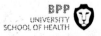

10. Red eye

Instructions to candidates

Name: Gary Walker
Age: 48 years old
Past medical history: Nil

Instructions to patients

Opening statement

> *I think I have an eye infection.*

Background
- You are a 48-year-old accountant and have attended today after noticing that your left eye has been red since you woke up this morning. The right eye is completely unaffected.

- There is a patch of redness next to the iris that was not there previously and has never happened before. You only noticed something was wrong when looking in the mirror.

- The left eye is slightly sore and uncomfortable but you would not describe the pain as deep or severe.

- You have not noticed any discharge from the eye and it does not feel itchy.

- There is no history of trauma or any foreign body to the eye.

- You wear glasses but have never tried wearing contact lenses.

- You have not noticed any visual disturbance and have not found bright light uncomfortable.

- There is no family history of eye problems (including glaucoma).

- From the red appearance you assume this is an infection and would like some eye drops from your doctor.

Data gathering, technical and assessment skills

History

- Unilateral or bilateral? – bilateral more likely to suggest viral or allergic conjunctivitis.

- Associated pain? – what is the nature of pain? (Deep or severe pain likely to require referral)

- Loss of visual acuity or any diplopia or photophobia?

- History of trauma to the eye or suspicion of foreign body?

- Discharge from the eye – more purulent in bacterial conjunctivitis; watery if viral conjunctivitis?

- Systemically unwell or any nausea or vomiting.

- Check patient's PMH and FH.

Red flags
- Decreased visual acuity

- Photophobia

- Deep pain as opposed to superficial discomfort of conjunctivitis or if pain is severe

- Sluggish pupil response

- Any corneal damage on fluorescein staining

- History of penetrating eye injury or of any chemical burn

Any of the above features warrant urgent referral for an Ophthalmology opinion to exclude more serious causes.

Examination

- Visual acuity – Snellen chart
- Pupil responses
- Ocular movements
- Examination of the eyelids and conjunctiva – presence of papillae, inflamed lid margins, eyelid swelling
- Preauricular lymph nodes
- Fluoroscein staining

Interpersonal skills

Ideas, concerns, expectations

- In this case, although your primary concern is to exclude serious pathology that may require referral it is important to know what the patient believes may be the cause.
- In this case as conjunctivitis is not the likely cause – and therefore, anti-bacterial drops are of no benefit – this needs to be explained in a context-appropriate way.
- Be sure to elicit other concerns as the patient may have other fears eg condition leading to blindness/being contagious.

Clinical management

History and examination are suggestive of **episcleritis.**

- Reassure and explain to the patient that this condition is not serious and will be self-limiting. However, appropriate safety-netting is also required.
- There are no red flags in the history and in this case it would be appropriate to manage with NSAIDs (if no contraindications to using NSAIDs from the history).
- Also try drops to soothe eye (eg Hyproemellose).

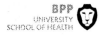

Safety net

- Advise the patient appropriately about red flag symptoms and need for urgency of assessment if these develop.

- Review after 48 hours if symptoms not improving as then an Ophthalmology opinion may be necessary.

- In all cases of red and painful eye keep in mind more serious pathology including acute glaucoma/iritis.

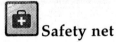

Further reading

1. Cronau H, Kankanala RR and Mauger T. Diagnosis and Management of Red Eye in Primary Care. *American Family Physician* 2010; 81(2): 137–144.

2. College of Optometrists (2015) *Episcleritis*. [Online]. Available at: www.college-optometrists.org/guidance/clinical -management-guidelines/episcleritis.html [Accessed 27 February 2017].

11. Low back pain

Instructions to candidates

Name: Rob Cooper
Age: 36 years old
Occupation: Scaffolder

Instructions to patients

Opening statement

I think it's my back. It's done in again.

Background

- You are Rob, a 36-year-old self-employed scaffolder.

- You have had low back pain for several days.

- This has been a frequent problem for you in the last few years.

- You have no symptoms in between each episode.

- You consider yourself to be fit and healthy otherwise and you attend the gym regularly.

- This episode of pain occurred while lifting heavy poles at work.

- The pain is located in your lower back and does not go into your legs. The pain is worse with movement.

- It is not affecting your sleep.

- You have had no problems with your bowels or bladder function.

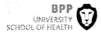
BPP
UNIVERSITY
SCHOOL OF HEALTH

- You have no numbness around your anus or 'back passage'.
- You have been taking paracetamol intermittently for the pain but this has not helped much.
- You have been unable to work for the last few days.
- You are concerned about how you will pay the bills if you remain off work.
- You are also worried that if these episodes continue you may be left crippled or in a wheelchair in later life.
- You are hoping that the doctor can recommend a 'scan' or some surgery that can cure the problem.

Examination findings of back

This is to be given to the candidate after they have performed an examination on the patient:

- No lumbar tenderness
- No deformity of spine visible
- Normal range of movement with pain throughout flexion and extension of lumbar spine
- Normal neurological exam of lower limbs

Data gathering, technical and assessment skills

History

- The patient's age and occupation will give you a good indication of a likely cause along with any circumstance of the episode.
- Age range 30–50 years old: the most likely causes are postural, prolapsed disc, degenerative and discitis.
- What are the circumstances of this episode? Has there been any injury or trauma?

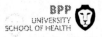

- Where is the pain located? Consider referred GI/GU causes of pain.

- How long has it been present?

- What are the triggers for the pain? Worse when resting and easing with movement suggests an inflammatory cause.

- Does the pain radiate anywhere else?

- Are there any neurological features eg numbness/weakness/sphincter disturbance?

- Ask specifically whether there is any past medical history of cancer, previous back problems/surgery.

Red flags
- Under 20 years old or more than 55 years old
- Non-mechanical pain
- Cancer or previous history of cancer
- HIV
- Prolonged corticosteroid use
- IVDU
- Weight loss
- Widespread neurological features

Yellow flags
Risks for developing and/or maintaining long-term pain and disability

- Belief that pain and activity are harmful
- 'Sickness behaviours' (like extended rest)
- Low or negative moods, social withdrawal
- Problems with claim and compensation
- History of back pain, time off, other claims
- Problems at work, poor job satisfaction
- Heavy work, unsociable hours
- Overprotective family or lack of support

> **Examination**
> - Assess gait
>
> - Examine lumbar spine movement – flexion/extension/lateral flexion/rotation
>
> - Examine lower limbs neurologically (including tone, power, reflexes, sensation)
>
> - Assess straight leg raise to check for nerve root irritation

Interpersonal skills
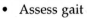

Ideas, concerns, expectations

- Identify the patient's beliefs about the causes of their pain as this will allow you to frame your explanation suitably and allow you to address management issues appropriately.

- It is necessary to find out the impact the condition this is having on the patient's life – eg ask about occupation. He may be self-employed or a carer and his primary concern may be regarding this rather than his own wellbeing.

    'How has your problem been affecting your life at home and at work?'

    'What were you hoping that could be done for you?' It is important to ask this as the patient may have unrealistic expectations particularly if his problems are chronic.

Consider using risk stratification (eg the STarT Back risk assessment tool) at first point of contact with a healthcare professional for each new episode of low back pain with or without sciatica to inform shared decision-making about stratified management.

Clinical management

The patient has an episode of acute mechanical low back pain.

- Explain the diagnosis to the patient relating this in a context appropriate for the patient.

- Reassure the patient that this will settle and not be likely to cause long-term consequences (which the patient may consider will be the case).

- Advise the patient to continue normal activity and reassure them that excessive 'bed-rest' is unhelpful.

- Inform the patient that further investigations are unnecessary for this type of problem.

- Start appropriate analgesia:
  - Consider NSAIDs if required, taking into account potential interactions and side effects. Use in conjunction with PPI if at increased risk of GI bleeding.
  - Prescribe oral NSAIDs at the minimum effective dose for shortest period of time.
  - Consider adding a weak opioid (with or without paracetamol) only if NSAID is contraindicated, not tolerated or ineffective.
  - Do not offer paracetamol alone to manage low back pain.
  - Do not routinely offer opioids for acute low back pain.
  - Do not offer opioids for chronic low back pain.
  - Do not offer selective serotonin reuptake inhibitors, serotonin norepinephrine reuptake inhibitors or tricyclic antidepressants for low back pain.
  - Do not offer anticonvulsants for low back pain.
  - If severely restricted movements of lower back due to muscle spasm – consider giving diazepam 2 mg tds for up to 3 days.

- Educate about future prevention including appropriate exercise/posture/lifting technique.

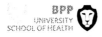

Pathology and diagnosis

- Back pain rarely represents serious pathology.

- Diagnosis is often difficult to establish but this does not prevent effective treatment.

- Acute back problems usually improve, but incompletely and they are likely to recur.

- Imaging is rarely helpful unless specific pathology is suspected or suspected surgery contemplated. Imaging of the lumbar spine for low risk patients can be overused given its low yield of useful findings, high yield of misleading findings, and lack of proved benefit for outcome.

- Physical activity and exercise does not cause damage.

Health beliefs

- Prolonged rest and time off work makes development of chronic, disabling back pain more likely.

- A positive attitude helps recovery.

- Complete abolition of pain is unlikely and maintaining a belief to the contrary can be a barrier to recovery.

Clinical management

- Find an enjoyable physical activity or formal exercise and do it regularly.

- Discomfort following activity is not a sign of treatment failure.

- Balance activity and rest.

Safety net

- If the pain continues to get worse, analgesia may need to be escalated.

- If symptoms are not improving, physiotherapy may be required.

- Advise the patient to return if any weakness of the lower limbs or sphincter disturbance develops.

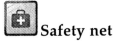 Further reading

1. NICE (2016) *Low back pain and sciatica in over 16s: assessment and management*. [Online]. Available at: www.nice.org.uk/guidance/ng59 [Accessed 28 February 2017].

2. Arthritis Research Council UK (2007) *Management of back pain in primary care*. [Online]. Available at: www.arthritisresearchuk.org/~/media/Files/Education/Hands-On/HO13-Oct-2007.ashx [Accessed 28 February 2017].

3. COST B13 Working Group (2006) *European guidelines for the management of acute nonspecific back pain in primary care*. [Online]. Available at: www.ncbi.nlm.nih.gov/pmc/articles/PMC3454540/pdf/586_2006_Article_1071.pdf [Accessed 28 February 2017].

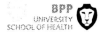

12. Tonsillectomy

Instructions to candidates

Name: Irfan Ahmad
Age: 6 years old

Instructions to patients

Opening statement

> *My son's throat is sore again.*

Background

- You are Nina Ahmad, a busy dentist with a six-year-old son (Irfan) whom you bring up alone.

- Irfan has had a sore throat for the last four days and you have had to miss work to look after him at home.

- You think his tonsils have become large again. He has a mild fever but no runny nose or cough. He says it hurts to swallow and has been eating less than usual since his sore throat started. He is drinking plenty of fluids and passing normal amounts of urine. He has no rash. He is otherwise well in himself.

- You are concerned at the number of days of school Irfan is missing due to recurrent episodes of a sore throat.

- Irfan has had four episodes of tonsillitis requiring antibiotics over the last two years. You have always tried to demand antibiotics from the doctors whenever he has been unwell as you feel this leads to a faster recovery.

- You have heard that a tonsillectomy will prevent any further sore throats and avoid Irfan missing any more school which will consequently make things easier for you to manage at work.

- Irfan's development as a child (eg speech, hearing, walking) has been normal to date.

- He has no drug allergies. There is no history of medical problems in the family.

Examination findings of child

This is to be given to the candidate after they have performed an examination on the patient:

- He is alert, looks well and is happily playing with the toys in your room.

- His temperature is 37.6°C. He has no rash or signs of meningism. He has moist mucous membranes.

- Respiratory rate is 20/min with no recession/tracheal tug. Chest is clear to auscultation. No stridor.

- Heart sounds are normal with no murmurs. Capillary refill time < 2 secs.

- Ear and throat exam – tympanic membranes normal. Tonsils are large, red and covered in pus. Bilateral tender, enlarged cervical lymph nodes palpable.

Data gathering, technical and assessment skills

History

- How many cases of tonsillitis requiring antibiotics have occurred in the past year?

- To what extent is this affecting the child's schooling? How much time off is he having from school?

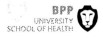

12. Tonsillectomy

- Are there any symptoms of sleep apnoea? – eg loud snoring, restless sleep, daytime somnolence.

- Any speech problems? – as this may be due to an underlying hearing problem.

Examination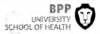
- General inspection – note alertness, hydration (eg moist mucous membranes, skin turgor), rash, photophobia.

- Vital signs – temperature, capillary refill time, respiratory rate, pulse rate.

- Any signs of respiratory distress? – tachypnoea, inter/ subcostal recession, tracheal tug, use of accessory muscles, nasal flaring, stridor/wheezing/grunting.

- Ears and throat – check tympanic membranes (if both are pink and inflamed then more likely to be viral infection). Check throat – if enlarged tonsils are covered in pus then more likely to be bacterial infection. Feel for any tender or enlarged cervical lymph nodes too.

Interpersonal skills

Ideas, concerns, expectations

- Explore the mother's understanding of tonsillitis and sore throats.

- What is her reason for wanting to arrange a tonsillectomy?

- Understand her concerns about the impact on her child missing school and the subsequent impact this has on her life.

- Her expectations are made clear however it is important to understand the motivation behind this.

Clinical management

- Reassure the mother that episodes of tonsillitis and sore throats are common in children.

    - Use Centor criteria when discussing risk of Group B haemolytic streptococcal infection and role of antibiotics

- It is usually unnecessary for any surgery except if the following criteria are met (based on Paradise Criteria – see 'Further Reading' below):

    - Impacting on school attendance

    - > 7 episodes in the last year or > 5 episodes per year for at least 2 years or > 3 episodes per year for 3 years

    - Airway obstruction resulting in sleep apnoea

    - Chronic tonsillitis

    - Recurrent quinsy

- Discuss risks of the procedure versus benefits to allow the mother to make a more informed decision.

Safety net

- Advise the mother that although her child does not require surgery at present (until meets Paradise criteria), a six-month period of watchful waiting to establish a pattern of symptoms (with review afterwards to reconsider tonsillectomy) can be adopted.

Further reading

1. SIGN (2010) *Management of sore throat and indications for tonsillectomy.* [Online]. Available at: www.sign.ac.uk/pdf/qrg117.pdf [Accessed 28 February 2017].

2. Paradise JL et al. Efficacy of tonsillectomy for recurrent throat infection in severely affected children. Results of parallel randomised and non-randomised clinical trials. *N Engl J Med* 1984; 310(11): 674–683.

3. NICE (2008) *Respiratory tract infections (self-limiting): antibiotic prescribing.* [Online]. Available at: www.nice.org.uk/guidance/cg69 [Accessed 28 February 2017].

13. Anxiety

Instructions to candidates

Name:	Tess Hunter
Age:	25 years old
Past medical history:	Nil
Occupation:	Legal secretary

Instructions to patients

Opening statement

> *I think I may be having a breakdown.*

Background

- You are a 25-year-old secretary who rarely attends the surgery.

- You have been experiencing a few alarming symptoms including poor sleep, feeling tense and wound-up.

- These symptoms have gradually worsened over the last year.

- At times you have felt panic in certain situations that you normally would have coped with.

- You work in a pressurised environment and have been finding it difficult to cope.

- You are embarrassed that you recently had a 'panic attack' at work in front of your bosses where you experienced chest pain and difficulty breathing with pins and needles in your hands and feet.

- These feelings of panic and a 'fear of going mad' are escalating and also affecting your social life.

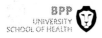

- You have not been in a relationship for some time and are finding it difficult to be around crowds and company.

- You have spent increasing amounts of time alone in your flat.

- You drink wine regularly and feel this may have increased to two bottles per week.

- You do not smoke and do not take other recreational drugs.

- You moved to this city just over a year ago and this is the first time you have lived so far away from family.

- You are close to your parents, but you have not been able to speak to them recently except on the telephone and do not want to burden them with your problems.

- You consider yourself to have always been a 'worrier'. However, you have only recently noticed this impacting on your life.

- You are afraid that you will have a 'breakdown' and that you will lose your hard-earned job unless you seek help.

Data gathering, technical and assessment skills

History

- Anxiety disorders range from simple phobias to generalised anxiety disorder.

- Psychological symptoms:
  - Panic
  - Feelings of unreality
  - Fear of losing control
  - Fear of going mad
  - Fear of dying
  - Worry
  - Tension
  - Inability to relax

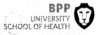

- Physical symptoms:
  - Pounding heart
  - Sweating
  - Trembling/shaking
  - Chest pains
  - Difficulty breathing
  - Dizziness
  - Nausea
  - Numbness
  - Tingling
  - Stomach pains
  - Headaches

- Duration of symptoms is important to differentiate causes. Generalised Anxiety Disorder (GAD) > 6 months often starts in adolescence.

- Nature of symptoms (eg episodic) to a definite trigger (eg phobia) or without any trigger.

- GAD more likely with concurrent over-arousal, irritability, poor concentration and poor sleep most of the time.

- Acute presentation can mimic other conditions so be aware of these:

  - Depression

  - Alcohol and drugs (including use of alcohol to control symptoms)

  - Psychosis

  - Post-traumatic stress disorder

  - Acute stress reaction

  - Iatrogenic

  - Physical – eg thyroid disease, asthma

- Previous similar symptoms? – age of onset

- What has she tried so far? – include any herbal options

13. Anxiety

- Assess risk factors for anxiety, such as:

  - Female
  - Family history
  - Life stresses
  - Personal loss
  - Poor social support
  - Poor health

> **Examination**
> - Assess for signs of thyroid disease.
> - Any evidence of delusions or hallucinations?

Interpersonal skills

Ideas, concerns, expectations

- Acknowledge the distressing nature of the patient's symptoms.

- Adopt a non-judgemental approach and also be sensitive when asking questions around psychosis, etc.

- Explore her thoughts about the cause of her worry and physical symptoms.

- Does the patient believe there is a physical cause or has she interpreted this as some form of mental illness?

- Consider precipitants for any 'panic attacks' – eg social phobia.

- Why has the patient attended today? Have her symptoms rapidly worsened?

- How are the symptoms affecting her life and ability to function?

- Is there a family history of similar conditions is she they worried that she will follow a similar outlook?

- What are her expectations about possible treatment?

Clinical management

- The patient is likely to be suffering with generalised anxiety disorder.

- Explain the nature of the condition – it is important to match this to the patient's health beliefs particularly explaining the link between physical and psychological symptoms.

- Reassure them that the condition is treatable and that they will be able to return to normal function.

- A step-wise management approach is recommended by NICE:

  - Grade severity using appropriate scale (eg Hospital Anxiety and Depression Scale (HAD)).

  - Identify possible triggers and avoid them (eg caffeine).

  - Benzodiazepines can be used in the acute phase however not recommended long-term (two to four weeks at most).

  - Self-help, information, support groups.

  - Cognitive behavioural therapy – explain to patient what this is and why it is likely to be effective.

  - SSRIs are effective and most appropriate first-line medication – discuss side effects, length of treatment and possible withdrawal effects before initiating therapy.

Safety net

- Follow up within two weeks of starting any medication or sooner depending on clinical situation.

- Only supply benzodiazepines short-term (but this would be after beta-blockers and other anxiolytics depending on the mutually negotiated management plan).

- Assess regularly to monitor effect of treatment.

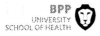

Further reading

1. NICE (2004) *Generalised anxiety disorder and panic disorder in adults: management*. [Online]. Available at: www.nice.org.uk/guidance/CG113 [Accessed 28 February 2017].

2. Simon C, Everitt H and van Dorp F (2009) *Oxford Handbook of General Practice*. 3rd edition. Oxford: Oxford University Press.

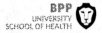

CSA Circuit 2

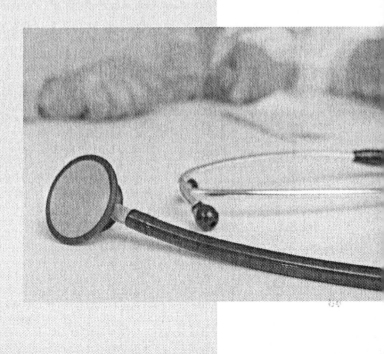

14. Depression

Instructions to candidates

Name: Alan Fullard
Age: 46 years old
Past medical history: Nil

Instructions to patients

Opening statement

> *I've been feeling very tired lately and I'm just not sleeping well.*

Background

- You are Alan Fullard, a 46-year-old accountant who was made redundant 2 months ago.

- You have been feeling low for the last six weeks.

- You live alone in your own home after your wife divorced you four years ago.

- You have two children that you have very little contact with since the divorce.

- Your social circle consisted mainly of work colleagues that you went to the pub with after work. However, since losing your job you cannot face being with them although they still invite you out regularly.

- You struggle to keep up with mortgage payments whilst out of work but have no other financial concerns.

- You used to play golf regularly but have stopped enjoying this recently.

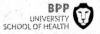

- You are finding it difficult to sleep and are often awake very early in the mornings, which makes you feel fatigued during the day.

- You realise that you have no motivation to look after your appearance and health as you should be.

- If you were working again, you think that life would be much better but you cannot see yourself getting employed again.

- You often wake up thinking 'what's the point?' but you have never thought of harming yourself.

- You drink every day, but no more than you previously did (about three cans of beer daily).

- Although you have not discussed your feelings with anyone else, you have attended today at the insistence of your mother who is very concerned about your lethargy and poor sleep.

- You would describe your mood as feeling 'a bit down', but you do not think you are 'depressed' and think that the term reflects weakness which only happens to other people.

Data gathering, technical and assessment skills

History

- Key symptoms for ICD-10 (International Statistical Classification of Disease and Related Health Problems (10th edition, http://apps.who.int/classifications/apps/icd/icd10online) criteria:
  - Persistent sadness or low mood
  - Loss of interests or pleasures
  - Fatigue or low energy

- If one or more of the above present for at least two weeks ask about other symptoms:
  - Disturbed sleep
  - Poor concentration
  - Low self-confidence or self-esteem

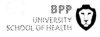

- Change in appetite
- Suicidal thoughts or acts
- Agitation or slowing of movements
- Sense of worthlessness, guilt, or self-blame
- Feelings of hopelessness

• Ask about any life events or precipitating factors eg at home or work.

• Past history of similar symptoms, psychiatric illness or chronic physical illness.

• Ask about alcohol and illicit drug use.

• Is there any family history of any depression, suicide or mental illness?

• Ask about level of social support – friends, family, work etc.

Red flags

• Assess suicide risk formally – there is no evidence that this increases the likelihood of self-harm and may, in fact, lower the risk.

• Need to document level of suicide risk in all cases of depression, especially if there are risk factors for self-harm.

• Does he feel that life's not worth living?

• Does he ever feel he'd be better off dead?

Examination

• Look for clues in appearance – eg self-neglect, strong smell of alcohol

• Flat affect

• Poor eye contact

• Monosyllabic responses or monotone voice

Interpersonal skills

Ideas, concerns, expectations

- Explore the patient's thoughts on their symptoms – maintain a non-judgemental approach as some patients may see the term 'depression' as stigmatising or they may just not have a cultural equivalent.

- Allow the patient to make the link between his symptoms and his life events/circumstances through reflection.

- Find out why the patient attended today – has he reached crisis point? Has he been encouraged by a concerned friend or relative?

- What are the patient's beliefs on how he can be helped – is he keen on starting medication? Does he see 'talking therapies' as a waste of time or vice versa?

Clinical management

- The patient in this case can be categorised as having moderate depression.

- This needs to be made clear to the patient in terms of simple explanation.

- Avoid collusion with the patient for fear of a stigmatising label, as only then can you tackle the problem.

- Tools such as the Patient Health Questionnaire (PHQ-9) and HAD score are useful to monitor treatment outcomes.

- The management options outlined below can be used in conjunction – discuss these with the patient and choose an appropriate strategy:

  - Leaflets/self-help advice (appropriate for mild depression)

  - Counselling – consider specific eg RELATE or CRUSE for specific causes

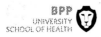

- Cognitive behavioural therapy – aimed at changing behaviour and coping strategies, effective with moderate depression

- Drug treatments (eg SSRIs):

  ○ No immediate effect for up to two weeks

  ○ Will be most effective after four to six weeks

  ○ Not addictive, but explain potential side effects, and discontinuation effects

  ○ Minimum total regime for at least six months

Safety net

- Review in two weeks (or sooner depending on clinical need).

- As not suicidal, it would be appropriate to give him one month's initial supply of SSRI.

- Consider seeing patient next time with a friend or family member that they feel comfortable with.

Further reading

1. NICE (2009) *Depression in adults: recognition and management.* [Online]. Available at: www.nice.org.uk/guidance/cg90 [Accessed 27 February 2017].

2. NICE CKS (2015) *Depression.* [Online]. Available at: https://cks.nice.org.uk/depression [Accessed 27 February 2017].

15. Benign prostatic hyperplasia

Instructions to candidates

Name:	Harry Hewell
Age:	68 years old
Past medical history:	Hypertension
Current medications:	Bendroflumethiazide 2.5 mg od
Blood tests from 2 months ago:	Sodium

Sodium	138 mmol/L
Potassium	4.0 mmol/L
Urea	5.7 mmol/L
Creatinine	99 mmol/L
Estimated glomerular filtration rate	> 90 ml/min

Instructions to patients

Opening statement

This is a bit embarrassing doctor... I'm having some trouble with my waterworks.

Background

- You are Harry Hewell, a 68-year-old retired foreman.

- You have been waking up several times at night to pass urine.

- This started over six months ago but is gradually getting worse.

- You have found that you have difficulty starting to urinate and that the stream is poor. However, you are passing good volumes of urine and you have no urinary incontinence. You have not seen any blood in your urine.

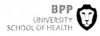

- It is at the insistence of your wife that you have attended today.

- Over the last few years, you have rarely attended the GP despite being on anti-hypertensive medication and you generally are non-compliant with treatment.

- You are embarrassed that you have to attend for such a sensitive issue and do not feel comfortable discussing this with a doctor whom you do not know very well.

- You have no systemic symptoms and are well in yourself other than these issues.

- You are worried that you may have cancer as a friend of yours was recently diagnosed after suffering similar problems although you have not mentioned your fear to anyone.

Data gathering, technical and assessment skills

History

- Ask about lower urinary tract symptoms – dysuria, frequency, urgency.

- Obstructive symptoms:

  - Hesitancy
  - Weak stream
  - Straining to void
  - Terminal dribbling
  - Incomplete emptying
  - Double voiding

- Irritative symptoms:

  - Nocturia
  - Daytime frequency
  - Urgency
  - Urge incontinence

- It is important to know about pre-existing sexual dysfunction as this can influence future management plan discussions.

- Other symptoms always worth specifically asking about:
  - Haematuria – consider other causes eg renal calculi, glomerulonephritis, cancer

  - Dysuria – any other symptoms/signs of sexually transmitted infections?

  - Polyuria/polydipsia – consider diabetes mellitus

  - Neurological symptoms

- Fluid intake including alcohol and caffeine

Red flags
Look for symptoms of malignancy:
- Weight loss
- Malaise
- Bone pain

Examination
- Abdominal examination

- Digital rectal examination – normally the prostate should be smooth and walnut-sized

- Urine dipstick

Interpersonal skills

Ideas, concerns, expectations

- Male patients may find certain subjects difficult to bring up and discuss with their doctor. It is important to recognise this and handle appropriately: 'I can see that you are uncomfortable talking about this, but this is a common problem and you have done the right thing to come and see me about it today.'

- Assess the impact this condition is having on his life.

- If you were to live the rest of your life with your urinary problem as it is now, how would you feel about it?

- Be prepared to discuss any erectile dysfunction problems openly and explain why it is necessary to know about this.

- Many patients with these symptoms will be worried that they have prostate cancer, so it is vital to ask him what he feels may be the cause of his symptoms.

- It is also important to explore other concerns and beliefs – eg would he ever consider surgery and what sort of treatment was he hoping for today?

Clinical management

- Discuss further investigations:

  - Mid-stream urine (MSU)

  - Prostate Specific Antigen (PSA) – it is important to discuss pros and cons of this test eg potential false positive result which will unnecessarily warrant further investigations

  - International Prostate Symptom Score (IPSS) – this is to assess severity and impact of urinary symptoms on a patient's life

- You need to be aware that the results of the above investigations may potentially guide you in a different direction (ie the diagnosis may not simply be BPH).

- Assuming that the PSA result is normal, explain that the likely cause for his symptoms is benign prostatic hyperplasia (or 'an enlarged prostate') and give a simple explanation about this.

- Reassure the patient that this does not increase risk of prostate cancer, but it can have complications.

- Discuss management options and reach agreed plan with the patient.

- Consider iatrogenic cause of LUTS; patient is on a diuretic, converting to alternative antihypertensive may be attempted.

- Consider 'watchful waiting' but remember to discuss coping strategies eg reduced fluid intake in evenings, reducing caffeine/alcohol intake, bladder retraining, urethral milking.

- Medical treatment including alpha blockers, 5 alpha reductase inhibitors, or a combination of both.

- Surgical options include transurethral resection of the prostate (TURP).

Safety net

- Red flag symptoms – development of these needs re-assessment

- Complications of BPH will also require review eg acute urinary retention

Further reading

1. Patient UK (2009) *Benign Prostatic Hyperplasia.* [Online]. Available at: http://patient.info/doctor/benign-prostatic -hyperplasia [Accessed 28 February 2017].

2. NICE CKS (2010) *LUTS in men.* [Online]. Available at: https://cks.nice.org.uk/luts-in-men [Accessed 27 February 2017].

3. Simon C, Everitt H and van Dorp F (2009) *Oxford Handbook of General Practice.* 3rd edition. Oxford: Oxford University Press. *Benign prostatic hypertrophy.*

4. Brown CT et al. Self management for men with lower urinary tract symptoms: randomised controlled trial. *BMJ* 2007; 334(7583):25. [Online]. Available at: www.ncbi.nlm.nih.gov/ pubmed/17118949 [Accessed 27 February 2017].

16. Dyspepsia

Instructions to candidates

Name:	Cyril Oates
Age:	37 years old
Occupation:	Bar worker
BMI:	34 kg/m^2

Instructions to patients

Opening statement

Can you give me anything for this terrible indigestion, doctor?

Background

- You are Cyril Oates, a 37-year-old bar worker.

- You have always suffered with 'indigestion' but, over the last four weeks, it has been increasing in severity and is putting you off your meals.

- You are experiencing an ache in your stomach, which is worse after eating.

- Your tummy tends to feel full easily and you always feel bloated.

- You are occasionally nauseous but have not had any vomiting.

- You have had no problems swallowing.

- You have not noticed any black stools or bleeding from your back passage.

- You have tried OTC antacid treatment (Gaviscon) but it no longer seems to help.

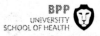
BPP
UNIVERSITY
SCHOOL OF HEALTH

- You have a busy lifestyle and have little routine – you have take-away meals often, as they are convenient (eg spicy curries).

- You smoke approximately 30 cigarettes per day and have never tried to quit (but you do want to stop smoking).

- You drink approximately 40 units of alcohol per week.

- You have recently put on 5 kg of weight and have stopped doing exercise.

- You have no relevant family history of stomach or bowel problems.

- You would like a 'cure' for your indigestion as it is now affecting your social life.

Data gathering, technical and assessment skills

History

- Enquire about symptoms – clarify exactly what the patient means by 'indigestion'

- Dyspepsia symptoms include:
    - Epigastric/retrosternal pain
    - Fullness
    - Bloating/wind
    - Heartburn
    - Nausea and vomiting

- Age of onset (see 'Red flags')

- Duration of symptom

- Measures already tried

- Risk factors:

    - Medication – eg NSAIDs, calcium channel antagonists, bisphosphonates

    - Smoking

- Caffeine
- Alcohol
- Obesity

Red flags
- Acute GI bleeding – warrants immediate referral
- Chronic GI bleeding
- Weight loss
- Dysphagia
- Persistent vomiting
- Iron deficiency anaemia
- Epigastric mass

Examination
- Examine for clinical anaemia (conjunctival pallor, pale palmar creases).

- If high alcohol intake, look for: jaundiced sclera, spider naevi, clubbing, liver flap.

- Examine abdomen for an epigastric mass or hepatosplenomegaly.

- Tongue – if red and enlarged (ie glossitis), consider iron deficiency anaemia.

- Check for lymphadenopathy (eg enlarged supraclavicular lymph nodes – Virchow's node on left side).

Interpersonal skills

Ideas, concerns, expectations

- Clarify the terms 'heartburn' and 'indigestion' as the patient may mean something very different.

- 'What do you think is causing your indigestion?' – check understanding of dyspepsia and see if the patient relates lifestyle factors to his symptoms.

- 'Are you worried it may be anything else?' – address his concerns and also be specific in your history about the occurrence of gastric cancer in the family.

- 'Has anything helped so far?' – has he made any lifestyle changes or tried OTC medication?

- 'What were you hoping I could do for you today?' – is he expecting to have any further tests? Is he looking for a tablet that will give him a 'cure'?

Clinical management

This patient has uninvestigated dyspepsia.

- Explain that this is a benign condition which can be effectively treated.

- Make the patient aware that certain aspects of his lifestyle are aggravating the situation.

- Give appropriate advice on how to make lifestyle changes eg healthy eating, smoking cessation advice, reducing alcohol/ caffeine intake, weight loss – 'exercise on prescription'.

- Continue antacids (but many would prescribe a proton-pump inhibitor (PPI) to allow his dyspepsia to settle).

- Further investigation is unnecessary in this case, but be aware of NICE guidance on two-week referral criteria.

- Consider endoscopy as routine referral in certain cases:
  - Previous gastric ulcer
  - Anxiety about cancer
  - Continuing need for NSAID treatment

- Assess response after one month.

- If lifestyle measures are ineffective, then add in full-dose PPI (eg lansoprazole 30 mg od) and re-assess in one month.

- Test and treat for H. pylori if there is no response or relapse. (There is no evidence currently whether to test and treat with PPI or to check H. pylori. A two-week 'wash-out' period is required where PPI must be stopped before checking H. pylori status.)

- Continue minimum dose of treatment necessary to alleviate symptoms on long-term basis.

 Safety net

- Once a measure has been implemented, arrange a review in one month to assess response.

- Advise the patient about red flag symptoms to ensure appropriate review.

- Ensure other members of the practice team are involved with preventative and lifestyle measures.

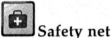 Further reading

1. NICE (2014) *Gastro-oesophageal reflux disease and dyspepsia: investigation and management*. [Online]. Available at: www.nice.org.uk/guidance/cg184 [Accessed 28 February 2017].

2. Simon C, Everitt H and van Dorp F (2009) *Oxford Clinical Handbook of General Practice*. 3rd edition. Oxford: Oxford University Press. *Dyspepsia*.

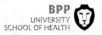

17. Diabetic review

Instructions to candidates

Name:	Rosie Best
Age:	57 years old
Past medical history:	Type 2 diabetes mellitus
	Hypertension
Current medications:	Bendroflumethiazide 2.5 mg od
	Ramipril 10 mg od
	Metformin 1 g bd
	Gliclazide 160 mg bd
	Simvastatin 40 mg nocte
BMI:	32 kg/m^2
BP:	128/80
HbA1c:	7.8% or 62 mmol/mol
	(Previous Hba1c 6.8% or 51 mmol/ mol 12 months ago)
Home blood glucose readings:	Range from 8.8–12.4 mmol/L pre-meals
Renal function:	eGFR 64 ml/min
	Creatinine 94 mmol/L
Cholesterol:	4.3 mmol/L
Triglycerides:	1.8 mmol/L
Retinal screening and foot check:	Completed with no issues

Instructions to patients

Opening statement

The diabetic nurse can't see me for two months and I'm due my review.

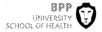

17. Diabetic review

Background

- You are Rosie Best, a 57-year-old school cleaner.

- You were diagnosed with Type 2 Diabetes three years ago and this is your annual review.

- You are very diligent at attending your reviews and are very compliant with your treatment.

- You struggle to lose weight and acknowledge that the dietary changes recommended to you have been difficult to implement.

- You saw a dietician when you were first diagnosed but the information seems more than a little hazy now.

- In particular, you have a 'sweet tooth' and find it difficult to give your treats up.

- Your job as a teaching assistant leaves you feeling tired at the end of each day and you do no regular form of exercise.

- You live with your disabled husband who requires a lot of care from you.

- You drive but do not do any long-distance driving and currently are not in the habit of checking blood glucose readings before driving.

- You do not smoke and drink approximately 20 units of alcohol per week.

- You have not experienced any side effects from your medications.

- Your fear is that you will end up needing insulin and the thought of self-injecting is terrifying to you.

Data gathering, technical and assessment skills

History

- It is difficult to address all the issues here in a ten-minute consultation unlike in surgery where longer time may be allocated for this sort of review. Therefore, it is important to tackle the main issue whilst acknowledging other areas that need to be addressed later.

- Ask about general wellbeing.

- Enquire about any specific issues regarding diabetes that the patient may have.

- Any medication issues? – side effects, hypos etc.

- Discuss education – have the following been addressed:
  - Diet
  - Exercise
  - Smoking
  - Alcohol

- Has the patient been seen by a dietitian or diabetic nurse or attended any structured group education?

- Is the patient up to date with annual foot and eye checks?

- Have the routine blood tests been done along with routine checks of BP/weight/urine dipstick?

Interpersonal skills

Ideas, concerns, expectations

- Are there any problems with your diabetes that you would like to discuss today?

- Consider depression in any chronic disease and screen for this.

- How is your diabetes affecting you?

- It can be very difficult to make so many changes to your life, how are you finding this?

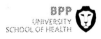

- Try to establish any specific concerns as well as if the lifestyle modifications and education are being optimised.

- You will need to reach a shared treatment target with the patient and therefore it is necessary to know the patient's opinion on further treatment and understand the impact on her life (eg job).

Clinical management

- Address the following areas:
    - Glycaemic control
    - Blood pressure control and overall CVD risk
    - Discuss blood results
    - Education
    - Medication – compliance

- Education should be reinforced at every review and should include:
    - Dietary advice

    - Exercise and weight loss advice

    - Smoking status

    - Ensuring foot and eye checks carried out

    - Involve the practice nurse/dietician and/or structured group programmes

- In this case, since blood pressure and lipid control are optimal, the primary issue is of lowering the HbA1c to within target range.

    - Discuss an appropriate target to aim for with the patient, tailored to their needs and circumstances.

    - NICE (2015) suggests HbA1c target of 6.5% (48 mmol/mol) for those on diet therapy alone +/- metformin.

    - If HbA1c increases to 7.5% (58 mmol/mol), consider dual therapy with:

- o Sulphonylureas (eg gliclazide, glimepiride)
- o SGLT-2 inhibitors (eg dapaglifozin, empaglifozin)
- There are four recommended options for those who require a third agent including: glitazones, DPP-4 inhibitors (or gliptins), insulin therapy or GLP-1 analogues.
  - o Glitazones (eg pioglitazone)
    - (a) Act by lowering insulin resistance
    - (b) Associated with increased risk of congestive cardiac failure and fluid retention
  - o DPP-4 inhibitors (eg sitagliptin, linagliptin)
    - (a) Inhibit glucagon synthesis which boosts insulin secretion
    - (b) Discontinue if < 0.5% decrease in HbA1c achieved after 6 months
  - o GLP-1 analogues (eg exenatide, liraglutide, lixisenatide)
    - (a) Increase insulin secretion, delays gastric emptying, promotes satiety and suppresses glucagon release after eating
    - (b) May be considered if BMI > 35 kg/m^2

- The choice should be made depending on patient choice/lifestyle and other co-morbidities.

- If HbA1c remains > 7.5% (58 mmol/mol), consider triple therapy with a licensed combination (eg metformin + DPP4 inhibitor + sulphonylurea; or a combination of metformin + sulphonylurea + SGLT-2 inhibitor).

- If triple therapy is not effective, not tolerated or contraindicated, consider metformin and GLP-1 analogue in patients with BMI > 35 kg/m^2. Adjust accordingly for ethnic groups. Discontinue after 6 months, if a reduction of 1% in HbA1c and weight loss of at least 3% is not achieved.

- Consider insulin therapies if HbA1c remains > 75 mmol/mol (9.0%).

- An example of an effective strategy for the management of Type 2 diabetes in a patient over 75 years old could be metformin (1st line) with the addition of possibly a DPP4 inhibitor (2nd line).

- See NICE 2015 guidance regarding blood pressure management, but aim for BP < 140/80 mmHg (but < 130/80 mmHg if there are kidney, eye or cardiovascular complications).

- Lipid modification for patients with Type 2 diabetes without CVD is to offer a statin if QRISK score is > 10%. Aim for a reduction of at least 40% in non-HDL cholesterol (NICE CG181).

Safety net

- Arrange a suitable follow-up review in appropriate time. If medication changes have been made, then review at three to six months as appropriate (HbA1c measures glycaemic control over the last three months).

- Warn about possible side effects of medication including hypos, weight gain, etc.

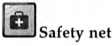**Further reading**

1. NICE (2015) *Type 2 diabetes: newer agents for blood glucose control in Type 2 diabetes*. [Online]. Available at: www.nice.org.uk/guidance/cg87/documents/type-2 -diabetes-newer-agents-final-scope2 [Accessed 28 February 2017].

2. National Collaborating Centre for Chronic Conditions (2008) *Type 2 diabetes: national clinical guideline for management in primary and secondary care (update)*. London: RCGP.

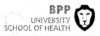

3. DVLA (2016) *Information for drivers with diabetes treated with non-insulin mediation, diet or both.* [Online]. Available at: www.gov. uk/government/uploads/system/uploads/attachment_data/ file/561792/inf188x2-information-for-drivers-with-diabetes -treated-by-non-insulin-medication-diet-or-both.pdf [Accessed 28 February 2017].

18. Palliative care

Instructions to candidates

Name:	Sam Beckett
Age:	59 years old
Past medical history:	Chronic obstructive pulmonary disease
Medications:	Seretide 250 Evohaler (fluticasone/salmeterol) 2 puffs bd
	Tiotropium inhaled powder 18 mcg od
	Co-codamol 30/500 2 tabs qds

Instructions to patients

Opening statement

I don't want to die in pain like my dad did.

Background

- You are Sam Beckett, a 59-year-old gardener who works for the council.

- One month ago, you started losing weight and coughing up blood and were referred urgently to a chest specialist. They said you had lung cancer, which was 'caught too late' as it had already spread to your liver and bones.

- You have come to see the GP with your wife as you have some concerns about how your lung cancer is going to affect you.

- You have smoked 40 cigarettes per the day for last 40 years, but quit when you were told you had lung cancer.

- You were diagnosed with COPD 10 years ago.

- You use two inhalers for your COPD: Seretide 250 (two puffs twice daily) and tiotropium (one puff daily).

- You also take co-codamol 30/500, 2 tabs 4 times daily, which adequately controls the pains in your bones from the cancer.

- Your father died from bowel cancer 20 years ago and you remember him being in extreme pain in his last few weeks of life.

- You are terrified you will also end up dying in pain during the terminal phase of your illness.

- You want reassurance from your GP that this will not be the case and you would like to know what options are available to you to ensure that this does not happen.

- You would also like to know what forms of support are available to you as someone living with cancer.

- If your GP can provide you with these things you will feel much better equipped to cope with your illness.

- You have no other medical problems in your family. You have no drug allergies.

- You have never worked with asbestos.

Data gathering, technical and assessment skills

History

- Ask him about how his lung cancer came to be diagnosed and if he had any risk factors that predisposed him to developing lung cancer (eg smoking history, occupation, history of asbestos exposure).

- Pain history – eg site, nature, severity, alleviating/aggravating factors, radiation, tried treatments.

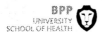

- Find out more about his COPD and how severe his breathlessness is and how it is affecting his life and daily activities.

Interpersonal skills

Ideas, concerns, expectations

- This case centres around Sam's ideas of the terminal phase of cancer based on his own personal experiences and his fears of exactly the same thing happening to him.

- The key is to explore his ideas of terminal cancer, dispel any myths and to reassure him that suffering from pain will not happen to him.

  - 'I understand all of your fears and concerns, but there are many things we can do nowadays to make sure your pain and other symptoms are well controlled.' It is important for him to tell you if his pain is not controlled and try to encourage an open dialogue.

  - 'There are also many support services available for both you and your wife that will guide and help you both through all stages of your illness.'

Clinical management

- Briefly discuss options of pain relief with him (as this is for the future), so he understands all the options potentially available:

  - Analgesia ladder: eg paracetamol, NSAID, codeine, tramadol, morphine.

  - Different formulations: eg tablets, patches, subcutaneous infusions.

BPP
UNIVERSITY
SCHOOL OF HEALTH

- Advise him to regularly update you if he feels that his pain is not being adequately controlled and then you can step up his analgesia appropriately.

• Support services available (and give patient contact details of them):

- Macmillan nurses can provide information to both patients and their carers about the different stages of cancer (and what to expect), the benefits they are entitled to and they can answer questions surrounding treatment options for various symptoms of cancer. They are often a good liaison service between the patient and their GP.

- For those with complex needs who wish to be treated at home, there are specialist palliative care teams who can provide intensive support at home ('Hospice at home'). These specialist multidisciplinary palliative care teams may include palliative care consultants and nurse specialists, physiotherapists, occupational therapists, pharmacists, dietitians, social workers and psychologists to provide holistic care to the patient.

- If you feel it is appropriate, this might be an opportune moment to discuss his end of life care preferences, such as preferred place of care, preferred place of death and DNAR status. But if you feel he is too worked up today, you may decide to review him again soon to discuss these issues when he is calmer.

Further reading

1. Macmillan Cancer Support. [Online]. Available at: www.macmillan.org.uk [Accessed 28 February 2017].

2. The Roy Castle Lung Cancer Foundation. [Online]. Available at: www.roycastle.org [Accessed 28 February 2017].

3. British Lung Foundation. [Online]. Available at: www.lunguk.org [Accessed 28 February 2017].

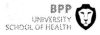

19. Migraine

Instructions to candidates

Name:	Rebecca Smith
Age:	26 years old
Past medical history:	Nil
Occupation:	Works in a bank

Instructions to patients

Opening statement

> *I have had these bad headaches and nothing is helping with the pain.*

Background

- You are Rebecca Smith, a 26-year-old woman who works in a bank.

- You have just been promoted and have been more stressed at work due to the increased workload and feel that you cannot take time off as you risk losing your job in these tough financial times.

- You are seeing the GP today as you started getting headaches four days ago and have had two episodes, each lasting about ten hours. They were both on the right side of your head and throbbing in nature.

- You feel nauseous during attacks but have no vomiting. You have had no visual problems but find that bright lights and loud noises make the headaches worse.

- The only thing you have found that helps is to go and lie down in your room in the dark when you have got home.

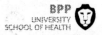

- The pain is 6/10 severity, but in between the headaches you are fine and have no symptoms.

- Regular paracetamol and ibuprofen have not helped.

- You are single, live on your own and are normally fit and well.

- You are not on any medications at present and have no drug allergies.

- There is no family history of note.

- You have done some reading on the internet and are concerned that it could be a brain tumour and so want reassurance from the GP that this is not the case. If you are not happy with the reassurance given to you, you will then ask to see a neurologist for a second opinion.

Examination findings
- Cranial nerves exam is normal.
- Cerebellar function is normal.
- Fundoscopy is normal.
- No photophobia and no neck stiffness. No scalp tenderness.
- Neurological examination of all four limbs is normal.
- Temperature is 36.8°C.
- Blood pressure is 118/72 mmHg.

Data gathering, technical and assessment skills
History
- Can she describe the headache pain? Ask specifically about the site, onset, character, radiation, associated factors, time, exacerbating/relieving factors, severity.

- Has she had any warning symptoms before it came on (auras) such as zigzag lines, dysphasia, hemiparesis?

19. Migraine

- Is she aware of any triggers to the headaches? Migraines can be associated with cheese, red wine, chocolate, caffeine, alcohol and stress.

- Find out what treatments she has tried so far and what effect they have had.

- Ask if she is on any other medications such as the combined oral contraceptive pill.

- Ask if this has happened before.

- Ask about her smoking status and alcohol intake.

- Ask if anyone in the family suffers with headaches or migraines.

Red flags

- Check to see if she has any symptoms of raised intracranial pressure such as a headache on waking or coughing and sneezing, or if there are any other focal neurological signs.

- A 'thunderclap' headache should be assessed urgently.

Examination

You should examine the following:

- Temperature

- Photophobia

- Blood pressure

- Fundoscopy – check for papilloedema

- Full neurological examination – this should include cranial nerves, cerebellar function and upper and lower limb neurology checking for tone, power, sensation and reflexes (especially if suggested by the history)

- Head and neck – scalp, neck muscles and temporal arteries

Interpersonal skills

Ideas, concerns, expectations

- You need to explore the reasons why she came to see you today and elicit her thoughts about what is going on and what her concerns are it could be – ie a brain tumour in this case. Brain tumours or meningitis can be common fears that arise from headaches. Patients may leave the consultation dissatisfied unless this concern is addressed and reassurance is provided. Does she know someone who has/had a brain tumour or has she read or seen something that has made her think about this? If so, then acknowledge this and reassure her that there is no evidence to suggest that this is the case with her.

- Find out what she is hoping to get out of seeing you today – is it other treatment for symptom control, is it further investigations or a specialist referral, or is it simply just some reassurance?

Clinical management

- Reassure her that this is a migraine and that there is no evidence of anything sinister like a brain tumour.

- Reassure her that there is no need to carry out any further investigations or for her to see a specialist at this stage. This may require some careful negotiation and if the patient is not happy after this, they will then insist on a neurology referral and if you cannot provide this, then they may see a specialist privately.

- Advise her to avoid any known triggers (in this case, stress at her workplace). Other triggers include: chocolate, cheese, citrus fruits, alcohol, missed meals, sleep (lack or excess of) and drugs (combined oral contraceptives and vasodilators). Some occur one to two days before start of menstruation.

- Advise her to keep a symptom diary over the next few weeks and try to find ways to relax more.

- Suggest trying something like Migraleve with an anti-emetic to see how she responds.

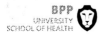
BPP
UNIVERSITY
SCHOOL OF HEALTH

- If she is not happy, you could start her on sumatriptan and explain how to take this – take one tablet at the start of an attack and repeat after two hours if needed.

- You could discuss prophylactic medications with her should the frequency of attacks increase (eg propranolol, amitryptiline).

- Give her verbal and written information on migraines.

- If there is enough time you could carry out the Migraine Disability Assessment Score (MIDAS) with her (see 'Further Reading').

Safety net

- Arrange to follow her up for review in a few weeks to determine the effectiveness of the treatment and to review her headache symptom diary.

- Advise her to come back sooner if symptoms worsening or if she develops any red flags.

- If any red flags present, then an urgent two-week wait referral would need to be done for a CT brain, or possibly calling 999 for an ambulance if symptoms suggest acutely raised intracranial pressure or a possible intracranial haemorrhage.

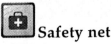
Further reading

1. BASH (2010) *Guidelines for All Healthcare Professionals in the Diagnosis and Management of Migraine, Tension-Type, Cluster and Medication-Overuse Headache*. [Online]. Available at: www.bash.org.uk/wp-content/uploads/2012/07/10102 -BASH-Guidelines-update-2_v5-1-indd.pdf [Accessed 18 February 2017].

2. NICE (2015) *Headaches In Over 12s: Diagnosis and management*. [Online]. Available at: www.nice.org.uk/guidance/cg150 [Accessed 18 February 2017].

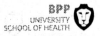

3. NICE CKS (2016) *Migraine*. [Online]. Available at: https://cks.nice.org.uk/migraine [Accessed 18 February 2017].

4. SIGN (2008) *Diagnosis and management of headaches in adults*. [Online]. Available at: www.sign.ac.uk/pdf/qrg107.pdf [Accessed 18 February 2017].

5. Stewart WF et al. Validity of the Migraine Disability Assessment (MIDAS) score in comparison to a diary-based measure in population sample of migraine sufferers. *Pain* 2000; 88(1):41-42. [Online]. Available at: www.bash.org.uk/wp-content/uploads/2012/07/MIDAS.pdf [Accessed 18 February 2017].

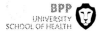

20. Alcohol misuse

Instructions to candidates

Name:	David Andrews
Age:	37 years old
Past medical history:	Nil
Social history:	Unemployed, divorced

Instructions to patients

Opening statement

> *I need help with my drinking.*

Background

- You are David Andrews, a 37-year-old man.

- You were divorced 3 months ago and your wife has taken your 12-year-old boy to live with her.

- You have been drinking more alcohol in order to cope with this. You have always drunk two to three pints of beer most nights but since the divorce you now also drink a bottle of vodka daily too.

- As a result you have lost your job as a security guard as you were found to be intoxicated at work.

- You want some help with your drinking and are happy to try anything.

- Your mood is low and you are not eating or sleeping very well at the moment. You have not had any thoughts about harming yourself or committing suicide. You have never suffered with depression before.

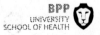
BPP
UNIVERSITY
SCHOOL OF HEALTH

- You have some close friends and family nearby and they have commented on your drinking before but you have got angry with them in the past about this.

- You are fit and well. You do not take any medications for anything.

- Your father used to be a heavy drinker but sadly he passed away a few years ago.

Data gathering, technical and assessment skills

History

- Ask this patient more details about his drinking such as the quantity, frequency, strength and type of drinks. Use the Alcohol Use Disorders Identification Test (AUDIT) questionnaire if available (can be more time consuming) or the CAGE questionnaire; these will enable you to assess his risk through drinking and his level of drinking. Please see 'Further reading' section.

- The AUDIT to identify his risk through drinking:
  - Low-risk drinking: score of 1–7
  - Hazardous drinking: score of 8–15
  - Harmful drinking: score of 16–19
  - Possible alcohol dependence: score of 20 or more

- CAGE questions enable you to assess his level of drinking:
  - Lower risk – this implies that no level of alcohol consumption is completely safe

  - Increasing risk – this involves regularly drinking more than 2–3 units for women and 3–4 units for men per day

  - Higher risk – this is regularly drinking more than 6 units per day for women or more than 8 units per day for men or more than 35 units per week for women and 50 units per week for men

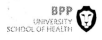

- Ask him if he has taken any other substances such as cocaine recently or in the past. Has he been known to mental health services in the past?

- Ask him about any risk of alcohol dependence such as a need to increase what he drinks to achieve the desired effect, an urge to drink, a lack of control, any withdrawal symptoms such as tremor.

- Ask him about his drinking behaviour in the past and how long he has drunk like this.

- Ask if he has had previous problems with his home life, work, driving and police due to alcohol.

- Ask him about his mood – check for symptoms of depression such as his sleep, appetite, weight, anhedonia, thoughts of self-harm or suicide. Carry out a PHQ-9 with him to get a baseline of his mood.

- Ask him more details about his relationship and the divorce and how he feels about this.

- Ask him about physical symptoms that could be related to alcohol such as vomiting (including haematemesis), weight changes, abdominal pains, tremors, confusion.

- Ask him how important it is for him to change his drinking. Use the 'Readiness Ruler' for this which uses a scale of one to ten (one being not important and ten being very important).

Examination

- Blood pressure
- Weight
- Breath – does he smell of alcohol?
- Tremor – is this a sign of withdrawal?
- Speech – is it dysarthric?
- Check for stigmata of liver disease – jaundice, gynaecomastia, spider naevi, ascites, palmar erythema, tremor, caput medusae, testicular atrophy, hepatomegaly

Interpersonal skills

Ideas, concerns, expectations

- Ask him if he knows what the safe limits of alcohol are.
- Ask him how his drinking is affecting his life, work and relationships. What does he want to do about this? What point in the stages of change cycle is he?
- What are his concerns – is there anything specific such as financial worries, relationships with his family or child, other social issues?
- Ask him what he would like you to provide him with today and in the future. Does he have hopes for a quick fix?
- Try to elicit his feelings such as low mood, guilt or worthlessness.
- Remember to be empathic and encourage self-efficacy. This is all more likely if you use a patient-centred approach. The most important aspect of the advice is to help him establish a goal to change his drinking behaviour.

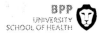

Clinical management

- If you feel the need arrange some blood tests – check the FBC (high MCV), LFT (high GGT in high ethanol intake and high ALT if liver impairment), glucose, U&Es, and INR (increase in liver failure).

- Explain to him the dangers of his drinking and explain what the recommended safe alcohol limits are. Educate him on the health benefits of reducing his alcohol such as lower blood pressure, reduced risk of stroke and heart disease.

- Offer him some brief intervention if he wants this. This involves providing him with feedback on his risk and highlighting his responsibility for change. Advise him on gradually reducing his alcohol intake and provide him with a menu of options for change, be empathetic and encourage self-efficacy (FRAMES structure for brief advice). This is all more likely if you use a patient-centred approach. The most important aspect of the advice is to help him establish a goal to change his drinking behaviour.

- Advise him not to drive if under the influence of alcohol.

- Give him information about Alcoholics Anonymous with possible to referral to local community alcohol detox or drugs and alcohol addiction services.

- Give him contact details for services such as Relate or offer referral to a counsellor if he wants to discuss things further regarding his divorce and mood.

- Suggest he starts medication such as vitamins B and C if appropriate.

- Consider detoxification if required with the community addiction team or yourself.

- Advise him to keep a diary of his alcohol consumption and agree on targets to try to achieve.

- Discuss that relapse is common and to give him support and encouragement.

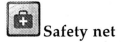 Safety net

- Arrange a review with him to assess the situation in terms of his mood and drinking.

- Encourage him to get support from family or friends and bring them along with him to the next appointment if he wants.

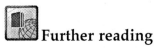 Further reading

1. Department of Health (2016) *UK Chief Medical Officer's Alcohol Guidelines Review: Summary of the Proposed Guidelines. January 2016.* [Online]. Available at: www.gov.uk/government/uploads/system/uploads/attachment_data/file/489795/summary.pdf [Accessed 18 February 2017].

2. NICE CKS (2015). *Alcohol – problem drinking.* [Online]. Available at: https://cks.nice.org.uk/alcohol-problem-drinking [Accessed 18 February 2017].

3. Babor TF, de la Fuente JR, Saunders J and Grant M (1989). *AUDIT: The alcohol use disorders identification test. Guidelines for use in primary health care.* [Online]. Available at: http://apps.who.int/iris/bitstream/10665/67205/1/WHO_MSD_MSB_01.6a.pdf [Accessed 18 February 2017].

4. Ewing JA. Detecting alcoholism: The CAGE questionnaire. *JAMA* 1984; 252 (14):1905–1907. [Online]. Available at: www.patient.co.uk/doctor/Alcohol-Use-Disorders-Identification-Test-%28AUDIT%29.htm [Accessed 18 February 2017].

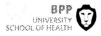

21. Carpal tunnel syndrome

Instructions to candidates

Name:	Amy Chung
Age:	38 years old
Past medical history:	Nil
Occupation:	Secretary

Instructions to patients

Opening statement

> *I have been having tingling and pain in both my hands.*

Background

- You are Amy Chung, a 38-year-old woman.

- You work as a secretary and have done so for the last 16 years.

- You have come to see the GP today as you have been having pain and tingling in your fingers in both hands for the last few months.

- It is the thumb, index, middle and half of your ring finger that are affected in both hands.

- Initially it was in the right hand only but is now both. It is worse at night and you find that shaking your hands relieves the symptoms.

- It is getting worse and is affecting you during the day at work and also at home when you are trying to pick up things.

- You are right handed and you have noticed you are dropping things in this hand because of the pain.

- You are worried about it being a serious problem.

- You suffer with hypothyroidism and are on levothyroxine tablets for this. You are well otherwise and are not on any other medications.

- You have three children and are happily married. Your husband has had a vasectomy as you both decided you did not want any more children.

Examination findings

This is to be given to the candidate after they have performed an examination on the patient:

- Bilateral tingling in the lateral three and a half fingers of both hands

- Weakness of thumb abduction in both hands

- Tinel's and Phalen's test are positive in both hands

Data gathering, technical and assessment skills

History

- Ask her about the pain and tingling – when did it start, what is it like, which fingers are affected, how often is it there, when is it worse, does anything make it better (is it better at weekends or holidays), how long does it last, any weakness in her hands (especially the thumb grip causing her to drop things)?

- Ask her about other changes in her hand such as any dry skin, colour changes or swelling in hand/along tendons.

- Ask her what treatment she has tried so far and if she has any allergies to anything.

- What is her occupation and what activities does it involve? How this been affected by her problem?

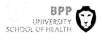

21. Carpal tunnel syndrome

- Ask her about any other medical problems, in view of carpal tunnel syndrome you should ask about rheumatoid arthritis, osteoarthritis, hypothyroidism, diabetes, acromegaly.

- Ask her if she uses contraception and if there is any chance she may be pregnant.

- Ask her if there is any family history of similar problems.

- Ask how much this is affecting her daily activities.

Red flags
- Check both her hands for thenar muscle wasting, if this is present then refer her urgently for surgical decompression.

Examination
- Check her weight as obesity is associated with carpal tunnel syndrome.

- Inspect her hands looking for any deformity, swellings, muscle wasting, skin changes or scars. Check her finger and wrist movements and power in her hand – pincer grip and power grip.

- Check the sensation in her hands.

- Check her thumb abduction.

- Check her palms for thenar muscle wasting.

- Carry out Tinel's test by tapping over the carpal tunnel in both her wrists to see if this elicits her tingling or pain.

- Carry out Phalen's test by hyperflexing her wrists to see if this triggers her symptoms.

Interpersonal skills

Ideas, concerns, expectations

- Ensure you ask what she is worried it could be and elicit her fear of it being something serious and worsening.

- Ask her what she is hoping you can do by seeing her today.

- Explain in simple terms what carpal tunnel syndrome is, any investigations that are needed and reassure her that it can be treated.

Clinical management

- If you feel it is needed then do some blood tests for FBC, U&Es, TFTs, ESR, CRP, fasting glucose. Arrange nerve conduction if diagnosis in doubt.

- Explain to her verbally what carpal tunnel is and provide her with an information leaflet on this.

- Advise her on conservative management initially – resting her hands and avoiding any precipitating factors – can try speaking to boss at work to look at ergonomics, use a wrist splint at night for both hands.

- Discuss the use of NSAIDs for the pain.

- Explore the options if these measures do not work such as use of steroid injections or surgery with carpal tunnel release.

- Decide together on a mutual time to review again to see if things have improved.

- If her symptoms remain the same or are worsening or she starts to have thenar muscle wasting, then refer her urgently for surgery.

21. Carpal tunnel syndrome

Safety net

- Arrange follow-up with her if symptoms worsen or do not improve with time, or just for a routine review.

Further reading

NICE CKS (2016) *Carpal tunnel syndrome*. [Online]. Available at: https://cks.nice.org.uk/carpal-tunnel-syndrome [Accessed 18 February 2017].

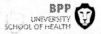

22. Deep vein thrombosis

Instructions to candidates

Name: Rachel Bolton
Age: 24 years old
Past medical history: Nil

Instructions to patients

Opening statement

I have got severe pain and swelling in my leg.

Background

- You are Rachel Bolton, a 24-year-old woman.

- You are visiting the doctor today as you developed pain and swelling in your right leg two days ago, which has got worse.

- You have not injured your leg in any way and have not had any surgery recently.

- You returned from your holiday in Australia three days ago.

- You work as a gym instructor and are normally fit and well.

- You are in a stable relationship and are on the combined contraceptive pill Microgynon.

- You are not on any other medications and are not allergic to anything.

- There is no history of any serious problems in the family including cancer, strokes and blood clots.

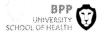

22. Deep vein thrombosis

- You are worried that you have got a clot in your leg from the flight. A friend had similar symptoms after they had an operation and you remember them telling you long flights can cause them.

- You want the GP to tell you what is wrong.

- You know that your friend had some injections for their blood clot. If you do have a clot, you are very anxious about the injections people have for this, as you are needle phobic.

- If the GP suggests possible treatment with injections, you can disclose your anxiety about needles to them.

Examination findings

This is to be given to the candidate after they have performed an examination on the patient:

- Vital signs are normal, oxygen saturations are 97% on air.

- The chest is clear to auscultation.

- Her right calf is red, hot and swollen. Right calf diameter is > 3 cm larger than that of the left calf. There are no signs of cellulitis. She has more pain on dorsiflexion of her right foot.

- Well's score for DVT is 2 ie high risk of DVT.

Data gathering, technical and assessment skills

History

- Ask her about the leg swelling and pain – when did it start, is it getting worse, where it started, is the area of the leg warm and red, is there anything that makes the symptoms worse or better, has she tried anything already for it?

- Ask her about symptoms of pulmonary embolism such as shortness of breath, cough or wheeze, haemoptysis or any pleuritic chest pain.

- Ask her about risk factors for DVT – has she had any previous DVT or PE, any recent surgery, has she been on a recent long-haul flight, any recent immobility, does she have a malignancy, is she taking the contraceptive pill?

- Has she had any trauma to the leg?

- Is there any possibility of pregnancy?

- Ask if she suffers with any other medical problems.

- Is she taking any other medications?

- Ask about her thoughts on what it is and her concerns.

Red flags
- If she has a DVT then she is at risk of PE also so you need to check for symptoms of this also.

Examination
- Inspect her leg for swelling and measure the calf circumference 10 cm below the tibial tuberosity and look for > 3 cm difference in calf circumference.

- Check her leg for pitting oedema in the right leg.

- Look for tenderness along entire deep vein system.

- Look for collateral superficial veins (non-varicose).

- Check for absence of signs pointing to an alternative diagnosis.

- Check for worsening pain on dorsiflexion of foot.

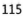

Interpersonal skills

Ideas, concerns, expectations

- Ask her what she thinks may be happening and elicit her concerns about this.

- Discuss the need to arrange further investigations and refer her to hospital for this. Discuss the management with her if there is a DVT. Explain what the 'injections' (ie low molecular weight heparin) are for and that they are short term only. Also explain that she will need to start warfarin or a NOAC for three months unless she has an underlying thrombotic tendency.

Clinical management

- From your history and examination assess her risk of having a DVT.

- Based upon her risk, explain the need to refer her for urgent further investigation and that this may involve blood tests and an ultrasound scan.

- Explain to her that if a DVT is confirmed then she will need heparin injections initially, but then will need to start warfarin or a NOAC and so the injections will only be for a short period.

- Advise her regarding doing exercises for her calves and keeping her leg elevated and wearing TED stockings.

- Advise her that she will need to stop her contraceptive pill and will therefore need to discuss future contraception later.

- Discuss she may need to have some screening after to check for cause if it is confirmed DVT.

 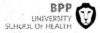

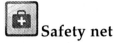 Safety net

- In this case, referral is needed acutely and so there is no safety-netting needed at present.

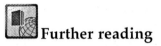 Further reading

1. NICE CKS (2013) *Deep vein thrombosis*. [Online]. Available at: https://cks.nice.org.uk/deep-vein-thrombosis [Accessed 18 February 2017].

2. NICE CKS (2016) *Anticoagulation – oral*. [Online]. Available at: https://cks.nice.org.uk/anticoagulation-oral [Accessed 18 February 2017].

3. SIGN (2010) *Prevention and management of venous thromboembolism*. [Online]. Available at: www.sign.ac.uk/pdf/qrg122.pdf [Accessed 18 February 2017].

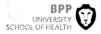

23. Multiple sclerosis

Instructions to candidates

Name:	Mr Brown
Age:	37 years old
Past medical history:	Nil
Occupation:	Retail manager

Instructions to patients

Opening statement

> *I just want you to check my eyes for me and tell me everything is ok.*

Background

- You are Mr Brown, a 37-year-old man. You have come to see the GP today because you have had some problems with your vision recently.

- You are actually very worried about this problem you had with your vision and are trying to get the doctor to agree that there is nothing to worry about.

- You started having blurring in the centre of your left eye a few weeks ago and it cleared on its own after a few days.

- There was no injury to your eye and your vision is normally fine and you do not wear glasses.

- Your right eye was fine and you have never had anything like this before. When moving your left eye it was painful.

- You have not had any other problems with your limbs or face such as weakness or headaches.

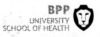

- If asked by the doctor you can remember several years back you had some tingling in your right hand which settled after a few days. You are otherwise fit and well.

- You do not take any medications for anything and have no known drug allergies.

- Your mother has diabetes mellitus and your father has angina.

- You live with your wife and three children. The eldest child is 18 years old and will be starting university later this year.

- You work as a manager of a large retail company and are worried that if it is multiple sclerosis then you will not be able to do your job properly and so your family will suffer financially. You also do not wish to be a burden to them.

- You are concerned that it is multiple sclerosis because you saw a recent programme on television about this and how it can often start with eye problems.

Data gathering, technical and assessment skills

History

- Explore his blurred vision in more detail:
  - When did he first notice it?
  - How did it progress?
  - Was there any injury to the eye?
  - Describe the blurring – any double vision?
  - Any associated eye pain, redness or swelling?
  - How did things resolve?
  - Any previous eye problems?

- Ask if he has had any other symptoms such as headaches, speech or swallowing problems, bowel or urinary problems, weakness or numbness in limbs or face, problems with balance.

- Has he had any similar problems like this before?

- Ask if he has any other medical problems or if there is a family history of any medical problems.

- Ask if he takes any medications and if he has any allergies.

- Ask him if he smokes and if he drinks alcohol.

- Ask him about the affect this has had on his work and home life.

Red flags
- If there is any acute focal neurology then he should be referred for further assessment the same day.

Examination
- Blood pressure

- Full neurological examination – assess the tone, power, sensation and reflexes in the upper and lower limbs. Check his gait and balance also

- Examine his cranial nerves

- Check for Lhermitte's phenomenon – flexion of the neck causes electrical sensation

- Fundoscopy – look for any optic disc atrophy

Interpersonal skills

Ideas, concerns, expectations

- Elicit his concerns about diagnosis of multiple sclerosis making sure not to disagree too much with his idea of it being nothing serious initially.

- Check if he has any concerns about his job or future problems.

- Check what his expectations are from seeing you today – does he want reassurance, further investigations or a referral?

Clinical management

- Explain the examination findings to him. Discuss how this episode and the previous episode of unexplained tingling in his right hand could be linked and should therefore be investigated further.

- Discuss that as the diagnosis remains unclear, he needs referral to a neurologist for further investigation. If asked by the patient about multiple sclerosis, you need to explain that it may be a possibility.

- Explain that he may have a MRI brain scan done and a lumbar puncture and some further eye tests. Explore his thoughts and feelings about this.

- Discuss with him about not driving until he sees the neurologist.

- You could arrange for some blood tests such as FBC, U&E, glucose and B12 and folate in the meantime and review with the results.

Safety net

- Advise him to come see you if any new symptoms occur before he is seen by the neurologist.

Further reading

1. NICE (2014) *Multiple sclerosis in adults: management.* [Online]. Available at: www.nice.org.uk/guidance/CG186 [Accessed 18 February 2017].

2. NICE CKS (2015) *Multiple sclerosis.* [Online]. Available at: https://cks.nice.org.uk/multiple-sclerosis [Accessed 18 February 2017].

3. DVLA (2016) *Medical rules for all drivers.* [Online]. Available at: www.gov.uk/driving-medical-conditions/telling-dvla -about-a-medical-condition-or-disability [Accessed 18 February 2017].

24. Contact dermatitis

Instructions to candidates

Name:	Helen Davies
Age:	42 years old
Past medical history:	Nil
Occupation:	Works in bakery

Instructions to patients

Opening statement

My hands have started to become sore and dry.

Background

- You are Helen Davies, a 42-year-old woman who works in bakery preparing the dough.

- You have only started working there a few weeks ago and since then you have been having patches of dry skin and soreness over your fingers on both hands.

- You have never had this before and so want to find out what it is.

- You think it could be related to the new job.

- You are fit and well otherwise and suffer with no medical problems.

- You are not on any medications and have no known allergies.

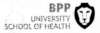

Examination findings
- This is to be given to the candidate after they have performed an examination on the patient.

- Red, dry, excoriated patches on both palms and fingers (which do not look infected).

Data gathering, technical and assessment skills
History
- When did she start her new job and what exactly does the job involve?

- What do her hands come in contact with at work?

- Does she wear gloves at work?

- What were her previous jobs and did she have similar problems then?

- Does she have the problem when not at work or on holiday?

- Has she tried any treatments already, and if so have they had any effect?

- Does she have any previous skin problems such as eczema or psoriasis?

- Does she suffer with any other medical problems?

- Does she have any thoughts about what it may be?

- Has she discussed anything with her boss?

Examination
- Check hands for signs of inflammation or infection – are there signs of scratching or itching, dermatitis, secondary infection?

Interpersonal skills

Ideas, concerns, expectations

- Check for her concerns, explain things clearly and ensure she understands.

- Ask her what she was hoping to get from seeing you today – treatment, referral or reassurance and advice.

Clinical management

- Explain the likely diagnosis to her of contact dermatitis.

- Suggest using some topic steroid cream (eg hydrocortisone 1% cream) and regular use of a medical emollient (eg Hydromol). Avoid using aqueous cream and E45 cream as these contain substances such as lanolin or sodium lauryl sulphate which can irritate the skin further.

- Explain to apply emollient liberally and to smooth into skin along line of hair growth. She must wait several minutes before applying topical steroid after this.

- Advise her on the use of gloves when handling the bread at work.

- Suggest that she discusses this issue with her boss to see if any other precautionary measures can be put in place there. Explain that if there is still no improvement after this or if her symptoms worsen then she may need to consider changing jobs.

- You could also discuss arranging for some patch testing to confirm the problem.

 Further reading

NICE CKS (2013) *Dermatitis – contact*. [Online]. Available at: https://cks.nice.org.uk/dermatitis-contact [Accessed 18 February 2017].

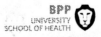

25. Menopause

Instructions to candidates

Name:	Julie Jones
Age:	54 years old
Past medical history:	Nil
Social history:	Secretary

Instructions to patients

Opening statement

I need help with my flushes, I just can't cope with them anymore.

Background

- You are Julie Jones, a 54-year-old woman who has come to discuss treatments for her menopausal symptoms.

- You have friends who are on HRT and so know a little about the risks with cancer but want this discussed further. You are open to other suggestions also.

- Your last period was two years ago.

- You do not have any urinary symptoms.

- You are up to date with your cervical smears and the last one a year ago was normal.

- Your husband has had a vasectomy in the past and so you are not on any contraception.

- You still work as a secretary in an office and your symptoms are starting to interfere with your work.

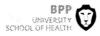

- You are also finding it more difficult to sleep due to your sweats and your husband has commented that your moods are getting worse.

- You are fit and well and you have not had any operations in the past.

- You are not on any medications and have no allergies.

- Your mother and sister have had breast cancer. Apart from this there are no other medical problems that run in the family.

- Your last mammogram was a few years ago and was normal. You check your breasts regularly and you have not discovered any lumps.

Examination findings

This is to be given to the candidate after they have performed an examination on the patient:

- Blood pressure 136/76 mmHg
- Pulse 78 bpm and regular
- Weight 70 kg

Data gathering, technical and assessment skills

History

- Ask her to discuss the symptoms she has been having – check for vaginal dryness, hot flushes, night sweats, mood problems, sleep problems, urinary symptoms. It may be worth starting a menopause diary.

- Ask her when her last menstrual period was and what her periods were like. Has she had any other bleeding since then?

- Is she up to date with her cervical smears and ask what the last result was.

- Is she using any contraception at present?

- Does she suffer with any medical problems? – in particular, any breast problems, gynaecological cancers, PE or DVT, strokes?

- Ask her when her mammogram was and what the result was.

- Ask about her family history – any blood tests clots in legs or chest, strokes, breast or gynaecological cancers?

- Ask her if she is on any medications. Ask if she has tried anything for her symptoms already.

- Ask her if she has any allergies.

- Ask if she smokes or drinks alcohol.

- Ask her what job she does and how this is being affected.

- Ask her about her home life and family and how it is affecting her at home.

Red flags
- Bleeding one year after last period, any irregular or painful periods, post-coital bleeding.

- Flushing with fevers and night sweats may indicate TB or lymphoma.

Examination
- Blood pressure

- Weight

- If any gynaecological symptoms then may need a PV examination

---

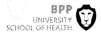

Interpersonal skills

Ideas, concerns, expectations

- Check the effect these symptoms are having on her life and check for symptoms of depression or anxiety.

- Find out what she knows already about HRT and the risks and other treatments.

Clinical management

- Discuss with her excluding other medical problems that may be causing symptoms such as thyroid disease.

- Advise her on lifestyle measures such as reducing her alcohol intake, stopping smoking, improving her diet, doing more weight bearing exercises, layering her clothing.

- Discuss herbal remedies with her such as red clover, sage, primrose oil, black cohosh.

- Discuss HRT and the different forms available (eg tablets, patches, creams). Specifically address the risks and benefits of HRT (in this case, with respect to her family history of breast cancer).

- Discuss other possible options such as SSRIs or clonidine.

- Offer to give her some more written information of HRT and also the other options discussed and to suggest she reads through them if she wants.

- Arrange follow-up with her for further discussion.

- If she decides she wants HRT, then review her in three months.

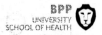

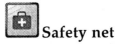

Safety net

- If she has any side effects on whatever treatment option she decides, advise her to come back to see you. If she has any other symptoms or worries to also come back.

Further reading

1. NICE CKS (2015) *Menopause*. [Online]. Available at: https://cks.nice.org.uk/menopause [Accessed 18 February 2017].

2. NICE (2015) *Menopause: Diagnosis and Management*. [Online]. Available at: www.nice.org.uk/guidance/ng23 [Accessed 18 February 2017].

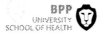

26. Seizure

Instructions to candidates

Name:	Mohammed Hussain
Age:	50 years old
Past medical history:	Nil
Social history:	Married with 3 children
Occupation:	Taxi driver

Instructions to patients

Opening statement

> *I never had anything like this before. I'm worried that it's epilepsy and that I'll lose my licence.*

Background

- You are Mohammed Hussain, a 50-year-old man who has had a seizure last night and has come to see the GP today.

- Your wife witnessed the event and has come with you as you cannot remember much of what happened.

- You were watching television and then suddenly you fell to the floor and your limbs were shaking and your eyes were rolled back. Your wife says that you also wet yourself which you are very embarrassed about. This all lasted three minutes and then stopped on its own. You were drowsy afterwards for a while (as if you were drunk) but then felt back to normal.

- You are very worried as this has never happened before and you do not want it to be anything serious.

- You are fit and well and not on any medications. You have no allergies.

- You have never drunk alcohol and you smoke two to three cigarettes per day.

- You are a taxi driver and your wife does not work as she looks after your three children. You are very worried about losing your driving licence as you know someone with epilepsy who had his licence taken away. You are concerned you will not be able to work or look after your family if this happens.

Examination findings

This is to be given to the candidate after they have performed an examination on the patient:

- Pulse 84 bpm and regular. Blood pressure 144/84 mmHg, with no postural drop

- Heart sounds normal

- Cranial nerves normal

- Cerebellar function normal. Gait normal

- Upper and lower limb neurology normal

Data gathering, technical and assessment skills

History

- You need to ask him and his wife more about the seizure – what happened before, what was he doing, any warning it was going to happen, what happened during the seizure, did he have any movement of his limbs, was there any tongue biting, was he incontinent, how long did it last, what happened afterwards, did he lose consciousness at any time?

- Ask him if this has happened before.

- Ask him how he has been since the seizure.

- Does he suffer with any other medical problems?

- Is there any family history of medical problems such as epilepsy, diabetes, strokes, sudden death?

26. Seizure

- Ask if he takes any medications at present or has any allergies.

- Ask him what his job is.

- Ask him what losing his licence will mean to him and his concerns.

- Ask him if he drinks alcohol or smokes.

Red flags
- First seizure, TIA, any focal neurology

Examination
- Pulse rate
- Blood pressure – both lying and standing
- Heart sounds
- Neurological exam

Interpersonal skills

Ideas, concerns, expectations

- Check his ideas about what he thinks it could be.

- Ask him about his concerns about what happened and about driving.

- Find out what he was expecting you to do for him.

- Explain that you will need to investigate further to find cause.

Clinical management

- Explain that this sounds like a seizure and as this is his first seizure there is a need to refer under the two-week wait for further assessment. Explain what this means to patient and what will happen in terms of when he will hear about his appointment and what test they may want to do.

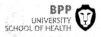

- Explain that he will need some further investigations to find out the cause – this includes blood tests for FBC, U&E, LFTs, lipids, glucose, TFTs, an ECG, EEG and an MRI scan.

- Discuss with him that he will need to avoid excess alcohol and sleep deprivation and also avoid any precipitants.

- Discuss safety issues like avoiding swimming or bathing alone.

- Explain to him that until he sees the neurologist he should not drive and that if he does drive, he will put himself and others at risk if he has another seizure.

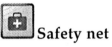**Safety net**

- Advise the family or carers of the person with suspected epilepsy how to recognise and manage a seizure and to record further episodes of possible seizures.

- Advise him to see you if he has further episodes.

Further reading

1. SIGN (2015) *Diagnosis and management of epilepsy in adults.* [Online]. Available at: www.sign.ac.uk/pdf/QRG143.pdf [Accessed 18 February 2017].

2. NICE (2016) *Epilepsies: diagnosis and management.* [Online]. Available at: www.nice.org.uk/guidance/cg137 [Accessed 18 February 2017].

3. DVLA (2016) *Assessing fitness to drive: a guide for medical professionals.* [Online]. Available at: www.gov.uk/guidance/assessing-fitness-to-drive-a-guide-for-medical-professionals [Accessed 18 February 2017].

26. Seizure

CSA Circuit 3

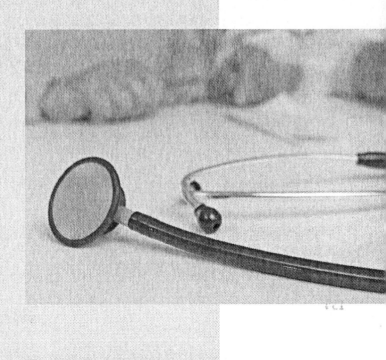

27. Antenatal care and genetics

Instructions to candidates

Name:	Jenny Smith
Age:	32 years old
Past medical history:	Appendicectomy
Occupation:	Receptionist

Instructions to patients

Opening statement

> *I'm pregnant and I'm worried my baby may have Down's Syndrome.*

Background

- You are a 32-year-old receptionist.

- You live with your husband, who works as a bank manager.

- You have been trying for a baby for the last six months and recently discovered that you are eight weeks pregnant and this is your first pregnancy.

- You are taking folic acid 400 micrograms daily and vitamin D 10 micrograms/day in a combined pregnancy multivitamin.

- You are aware about pregnancy advice with regards to diet/alcohol/smoking/cat litter etc as your sister told you about these, and if the doctor brings this up you move the consultation on.

- Your sister (aged 38) is also pregnant and has just had an amniocentesis and been told the baby has Down's syndrome. This is also your sister's first pregnancy.

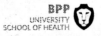

- You understand that Down's syndrome causes learning difficulties and the person to 'look different'.

- You want to learn more about Down's syndrome – what causes it? You have heard it is genetic – does that mean your child might be affected? Can you have an amniocentesis to find out?

- You know that an amniocentesis is where some amniotic fluid is removed with a needle and then analysed. You were not aware of the screening tests before this and that amniocentesis is only available to women who are at high risk.

- If asked, you were also not aware that there was a risk of miscarriage with the amniocentesis and you would not be willing to take this risk.

- If the doctor mentions the screening tests and explains them clearly, you feel that it is a big decision to make and you would like to discuss this with your husband. If the doctor doesn't explain the screening process clearly, you leave confused about why you can't go straight for amniocentesis.

- If the doctor asks what you would do if you found out your child had Down's syndrome, you would like to continue with the pregnancy. You therefore feel that there may not be any need to have any screening tests, but would like to discuss this further with your husband.

Data gathering, technical and assessment skills

History

- Establish more about the pregnancy – how many weeks pregnant is she? Was it a planned/wanted pregnancy? How does she feel now she has found out she is pregnant?

- Invite her to book in with the midwife.

- Ask about pregnancy health – folic acid/vitamin D/alcohol/smoking/cat litter/properly cooked eggs – ie health promotion advice.

- Why is she worried about Down's syndrome – explore her understanding of Down's syndrome – what does she know about it already? What would she do if she found out her baby had Down's syndrome – would it change her outcome of the pregnancy?

- What does she understand about amniocentesis? Does she know what is involved or what the risks of this procedure are?

Interpersonal skills

Ideas, concerns, expectations

- What is her understanding of Down's syndrome? Explore what she already knows and what she wants to know about Down's syndrome – remember this exam isn't about reeling off all that you know about the condition, it is about understanding the patient's agenda.

- What does a diagnosis of Down's syndrome mean to her and her husband? What would be the consequences of a high risk screening result? What would be the consequences of having a child with Down's syndrome?

- Her expectation is to have an amniocentesis – explore with her how she feels about this now she has more information. Has this changed her expectation?

Clinical management

- There are three core features of this case:

  1. General pregnancy care and advice (folic acid etc)

  2. Understanding and explanation of antenatal screening programme

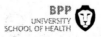

3. Understanding and explanation of genetic basis for Down's syndrome

- It may be difficult to cover all three in your ten-minute station; this is where understanding the patient's concerns and expectations is important to guide the consultation and to prioritise tasks.

- Acknowledging general pregnancy advice (smoking, folic acid etc) is always useful in a pregnancy case and shows evidence of health promotion.

- Explain that Down's syndrome is a genetic condition where there is an extra 'building block' in the person's genetic makeup.

- Explain the screening process for Down's syndrome: current screening in the UK is from 11 weeks +0 days to 13 weeks +6 days for the combined test (nuchal translucency and triple blood test). After this, the quadruple blood test can be used up to 20 weeks +0 days.

- It is important to explain that this is a screening test and is not diagnostic, meaning it calculates a risk of the baby being affected by one of these three conditions. A 'negative' screen does not rule out Down's syndrome.

- If the risk is > 1/150, it is deemed 'high risk' and then amniocentesis or chorionic villous sampling (CVS) is offered.

- These are both invasive procedures, which both carry a 1% risk of miscarriage.

- If the patient wants to know more about amniocentesis, you could explain that it is a procedure carried out at the hospital, where a needle is inserted through the tummy into the amniotic fluid (the fluid surrounding the baby) in order to take a sample of this fluid, which can then be analysed for genetic conditions and infections.

- Explain that Down's syndrome is genetic but is not an inherited condition. This is because the vast majority of cases occur

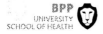

from non-dysjunction at meiosis – practising explaining this and the different modes of inheritance is useful as it can be quite difficult to explain this in layman terms. 'Each person is made up of pairs of building blocks; one copy of this pair comes from the mother and one copy from the father. In Down's syndrome an extra copy comes from the mother resulting in three copies of this set of building blocks. This results in Down's syndrome' is an example of how this can be explained. Some candidates like to draw diagrams.

- The risk of Down's syndrome does increase with increasing maternal age.

- Explain that Down's syndrome can present differently; there are characteristic facial features and all children will have some degree of intellectual disability. There are other health concerns including heart disease, hearing problems, visual problems (eg cataracts) and GI problems (eg duodenal atresia).

- You need to communicate with this lady that she would not be referred for amniocentesis unless her screening showed a high-risk result. You will therefore need to discuss screening and Down's syndrome and explore with her what her wishes are, now that she has this information.

 Safety net

- Providing the patient with a leaflet about antenatal screening and Down's syndrome would be useful. When giving an information leaflet, it is important to state what the leaflet covers, eg 'Here's a leaflet that discusses the screening programme for Down's syndrome and what Down's syndrome is', which shows that you have an understanding of why you are giving the leaflet, rather than a blanket statement of 'Here's a leaflet'.

- Then invite her to return, perhaps with her husband to discuss any other concerns, particularly any questions that may arise after reading the information.

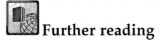

Further reading

1. NICE (2017) *Antenatal care for uncomplicated pregnancies.* [Online]. Available at: www.nice.org.uk/guidance/cg62 [Accessed 5 February 2017].

2. Down's Syndrome Association. [Online]. Available at: www.downs-syndrome.org.uk [Accessed 5 February 2017].

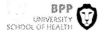

28. Anaemia

Instructions to candidates

Name:	Albert Finder
Age:	88 years old
Past medical history:	Hypertension
	Hypercholesterolaemia
	Gout
	Severe hearing impairment
Medication:	Amlodipine 10 mg od
	Ramipril 2.5 mg od
	Atorvastatin 10 mg nocte

Two weeks ago, Albert had blood tests done and the results are shown below:

	2 weeks ago	1 year ago	
Hb	9.7 g/dL	13.1 g/dL	(13 – 18 g/dL)
MCV	56 fL	80 fL	(80 – 100 fL)
MCH	20 pg	30 pg	(27 – 33 pg)
Platelets	210×10^9/L	233×10^9/L	$(150 – 400 \times 10^9$/L)
WCC	7×10^9/L	8.2×10^9/L	$(4 – 11 \times 10^9$/L)
Ferritin	7 ng/ml	18 ng/ml	(15 – 200 ng/ml)

Instructions to patients

Opening statement

> *I've come for my test results Doc.*

Background

- You are an 89-year-old retired engineer.

- You live alone after your wife died following a stroke two years ago.

- You have a daughter and three grandchildren who live nearby.

- You saw the nurse for a routine check up two weeks ago and came in for your blood results.

- You are severely hearing impaired, and if the doctor does not speak clearly and check that you can hear them properly, then you will nod along and look blank.

- You feel 'fit as a fiddle' and are surprised when the doctor informs you that you are anaemic.

- You have a healthy appetite, and your daughter pre-prepares your meals and brings them round to you on alternate days. She also does your food shopping for you. Your diet is varied with red meat on average twice a week.

- You manage well on your own at home with self-care etc and if the doctor discusses getting you extra support, you decline this at present, but may be willing to discuss this again with your daughter present.

- You have no upper or lower GI symptoms when asked (no change in bowels/rectal bleeding/tenesmus/dyspepsia/dysphagia/abdominal pain).

- If asked, you think you may have lost some weight as your trousers are a little looser, but you haven't weighed yourself recently.

- You have no history of overt blood loss.

- If asked, you are not symptomatic with respect to the anaemia (no shortness of breath/dizziness/palpitations/chest pain/fatigue).

- You have never had anaemia previously.

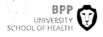

- There is no family history of blood disorders.

- If the doctor explains clearly what anaemia means, you wonder if this can be addressed by dietary changes. You are not keen on any medication.

- If the doctor is sensitive about addressing the need for urgent investigations and the possibility of an underlying malignancy, you will accept the tests and ask the doctor to inform your daughter.

- If, however, the doctor does not bring up the possibility of malignancy in a sensitive manner, you will become upset and disengage.

- You agree to have investigations done if the doctor explains clearly what they are in layman terms.

- If the doctor uses excessive jargon, you will become confused and refuse further investigations.

Data gathering, technical and assessment skills

History

- Ask about why he had blood tests done. Was it a routine blood test or to investigate any particular symptoms?

- The blood results show a new microcytic, hypochromic anaemia – you need to try to establish a cause for this.

- Has he had any visible blood loss?

- Has he had any lower GI symptoms – change in bowel habit/ PR bleeding/abdominal pain?

- Has he had any upper GI symptoms – dyspepsia/dysphagia/ vomiting?

- Has he got any constitutional symptoms – weight loss/ sweats? (If he does report weight loss, try to quantify this.)

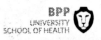

- Has he ever been told he has anaemia previously? If so, was this investigated and how was it managed?

- Is he symptomatic with regards to the anaemia – does he have any dizzy spells/light-headedness/fatigue/lethargy? Any chest pain/SOB/palpitations?

Examination
- Abdominal examination to assess for any masses or organomegaly.

- If there is any history of rectal bleeding or altered bowel habits then a rectal examination is warranted.

- If symptomatic with regards to anaemia examine sitting and standing blood pressure, pulse rate, auscultate heart for murmurs – looking for signs of decompensation.

Interpersonal skills

Ideas, concerns, expectations

- It is important to establish what his thoughts are about iron deficiency anaemia. Is this a term he understands? What does this mean to him?

- It is also important to explore what his thoughts are about investigations for potential malignancy – does he know what colonoscopy/endoscopy involves? What would the consequences be for him if they uncovered a malignancy? Does he have any worries when you talk to him about malignancy and the investigations and processes involved?

- It is also mentioned in the history that he is hearing impaired. In the CSA, there may be a case where a patient has a disability – this may be hearing or visual impairment, or they may be in a wheelchair, for example. It is useful to practise these in your group.

- In cases of hearing or visual impairment it is important to check the preferred method of communication early in the consultation and check understanding.

Clinical management

- These blood results show a new microcytic, hypochromic anaemia with a low ferritin. This is a picture of iron deficiency anaemia.

- Explain what this means without using jargon.

- The candidate should therefore explore possible causes for this, including overt blood loss, haematological disorders and GI malignancy.

- Overt blood loss can be established from the history.

- This gentleman states that he has a varied diet, so a dietary cause is unlikely in this case (and should be a diagnosis of exclusion).

- A haematological disorder would likely have presented earlier in life, or be suggested by a family history (eg thalassemia).

- As there is no obvious cause to explain the anaemia, he would warrant urgent (two-week wait) referral for suspected GI cancer. This, therefore, requires knowledge of guidelines for investigation of iron deficiency anaemia, and suspected cancer guidelines.

- It is important to explain to the patient that iron deficiency anaemia may represent an underlying malignancy and the urgent referral is needed to investigate this possibility.

- This patient would require a colonoscopy and gastroscopy to investigate for a possible underlying GI tract cancer.

- The process of the two-week wait needs to be explained to the patient; they may be seen in clinic first or they may go directly for gastroscopy/colonoscopy. At this stage, if any masses are seen, then a biopsy can be taken at the time of the test. It is useful to practise explaining this to patients.

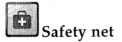

Safety net

- Important to inform the patient that they should expect an appointment within two weeks; if this does not happen then advise them to call the surgery.

- Invite the patient to return, perhaps with his daughter to discuss any further questions that may arise, or after his appointment at the hospital to discuss their investigative pathway.

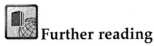

Further reading

1. NICE CKS (2013) *Anaemia – iron deficiency*. [Online]. Available at: http://cks.nice.org.uk/anaemia-iron-deficiency [Accessed 5 February 2017].

2. NHS Choices (2016) *Iron deficiency anaemia*. [Online]. Available at: www.nhs.uk/conditions/Anaemia-iron-deficiency-/Pages/Introduction.aspx [Accessed 5 February 2017].

3. NICE CKS (2015) *Gastrointestinal tract (lower) cancers – recognition and referral*. [Online]. Available at: https://cks.nice.org.uk/gastrointestinal-tract-lower-cancers-recognition-and-referral [Accessed 5 February 2017].

4. NICE CKS (2015) *Gastrointestinal tract (upper) cancers – recognition and referral*. [Online]. Available at: https://cks.nice.org.uk/gastrointestinal-tract-upper-cancers-recognition-and-referral [Accessed 5 February 2017].

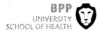

29. Domestic abuse

Instructions to candidates

Name:	Daniel Broad
Age:	35 years old
Past medical history:	Depression
	Five consultations over last three months with sore throat, thickened toenails, rhinorrhoea, wrist pain, ear pain. On each consultation, no red flags or abnormalities were found and patient was reassured.
Medication:	Citalopram 10 mg od
Social history:	Works as sales assistant
	Lives with partner

Instructions to patients

Opening statement

> *I need some more of my medication, and wonder if I can be entitled to free prescriptions.*

Background

- You are a 35-year-old sales assistant.

- You live with your partner, Mark, who is a sales manager at another store.

- You rent an apartment with your partner.

- You were diagnosed with depression 2 years ago and feel that the citalopram initially helped, but in the last 12 months you feel low again.

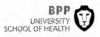

- You have never had any thoughts of self-harm or suicide, and no thoughts of harm to others.

- Your concentration levels are normal and you have no problems with your sleep.

- Your appetite and weight are stable.

- If asked about hobbies or activities you enjoy, you state that you aren't able to go out and see your friends. You used to enjoy playing squash regularly but aren't able to any more.

- If the doctor enquires further about why you aren't able to enjoy playing squash you reluctantly tell them that your partner wouldn't like it.

- If the doctor asks more about this in a sensitive manner, you explain that your partner becomes jealous if he sees you meeting friends without him, and he manages the finances so that you don't have enough money to go out and do things without him.

- You are given a spending allowance each week by Mark, and you can afford your prescription, but if you were entitled to free prescriptions this would allow you some spare money to start playing squash again with your friends.

- You have been with your partner for 5 years, and initially the relationship was good, but in the last 12 months, Mark has become more controlling.

- If asked, he has never been sexually or physically violent.

- If asked, you have no children and neither does your partner.

- If the doctor uncovers the issues in your relationship you reveal that you would like to end the relationship, but you don't feel in a financially secure place to do so.

- If the doctor doesn't uncover the issues in a sensitive manner, you will not reveal the information about control of money and that your partner doesn't allow you to go out with your friends.

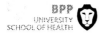

- If the doctor suggests that you are a victim of domestic abuse (financial and emotional) in a sensitive manner, you will consider help but decline it at present. But if the doctor seems dismissive of the subject then you will deny that there is a problem and end the consultation.

- If the doctor suggests follow-up, you will accept this and will consider your need for help or a helpline number in the meantime.

- If the doctor explains that you do not fit the criteria for a payment exemption certificate or is unsure but will look it up, you accept this explanation. If they offer you payment exemption you will happily accept it. However, if they do not address the issue you will raise it again at the end of the consultation.

Data gathering, technical and assessment skills

History

- Ask about his mood and other symptoms of depression:

  - How is his sleep? How is his concentration?

  - How is his appetite? Has he lost any weight?

  - What are his energy levels like?

  - Does he still get enjoyment out of activities? What are his hobbies?

  - Does he still manage to get enjoyment out of the things he used to?

- Is he compliant with his medication?

- Is he having any side effects from his medication?

- It is always important to ask with any mental health review about risk to self and others:

BPP
UNIVERSITY
SCHOOL OF HEALTH

- 'Do you ever feel that life is not worth living?'

- 'Have you ever had any thoughts of harming yourself?'

- 'Sometimes, when people are feeling low they have thoughts of harming others around them, has this ever happened to you?'

- When he mentions that he isn't able to go out and enjoy the things he used to, this is a cue. It is important to pick up on this and explore further:

  - Why isn't he able to go out like he used to?
  - How does he feel about this?
  - How is this affecting the relationship?
  - Is this impacting on his mood?

- If you learn about the domestic abuse, ask what his thoughts are about it – does he recognise that what is happening to him is classed as abuse? What does he want to do about the relationship?

  Note. If he has capacity and is not a vulnerable adult, his decision about further action has to be respected.

Red flags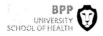
- Are there any children involved?

- Does this gentleman have capacity – if so, and he declines help, you have to respect this. If he lacks capacity, you will need to act in his best interests.

Interpersonal skills

- In mental health cases it is important to pick up on body language:

  - 'I can see you look slightly anxious when talking about this…'

  - 'I can see this is worrying you, could you tell me a little more…'

This will show the examiner that you are carrying out a mental state examination and picking up on cues, as well as guide the consultation and show the patient that you are actively listening.

Ideas, concerns, expectations

- It is important to establish why this patient feels they are entitled to payment exemption.

- What would be the consequences if they weren't entitled to payment exemption?

- Check if there was anything else they were hoping for from today's consultation, or was it just the prescription payment exemption? This shows that you have listened to him clearly expressing his expectations at the opening of the consultation, but are aware there may be other needs.

- When you have uncovered the domestic abuse, explore his thoughts on this:

  - Does he recognise this as abuse? How does this make him feel?

  - Does he feel that anything needs to be done about this?

  - How would he like you to help him?

Clinical management

- There are three components to this consultation: a medication review, a depression review, and establishing why he is requesting free prescriptions.

- In this instance, where a few issues are raised it is important to explore the patient's agenda to establish what is going to constitute the bulk of the consultation.

- It is unlikely that you will cover all three issues in this consultation. However, it is important to cover the red flags and acknowledge the three issues, to show the patient (and the examiner!) both that you are aware there is more than one issue and they will be covered, and that you can prioritise tasks appropriately.

- You will need to explore with the patient what he would like to do about this, if anything.

- Patients with repeated attendances for minor illnesses should raise the possibility of underlying mental health issues or domestic abuse.

- It is important in this consultation to explore what the patient feels is the problem and explore how he feels this can be addressed. You can offer resources available but, if the patient has capacity, it is their decision on further actions.

- It is important to remember that domestic abuse can be experienced by men, and in both heterosexual and homosexual relationships.

- Domestic abuse comes in the form of physical, sexual, emotional, financial and psychological abuse. It may be useful to explain this to the patient.

- It is important to ask about other forms of domestic abuse.

- Establish if there is any immediate risk, and (red flag) any risk to children. If there is, then the police need to be involved and child safeguarding procedures started.

- There is a list of services available to help victims of domestic abuse. You can signpost the patient towards the relevant agency:

  - 24-hour National Violence Helpline

  - Women's Aid

  - Mankind Initiative (for male victims of domestic abuse)

  - Broken Rainbow (for gay, lesbian, bisexual and transgender abuse)

  - Men's Advice Line

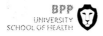

Safety net

- Offer to follow this patient up in a couple of weeks to monitor his mental health. This will also give him the opportunity to consider the information you have given him.

- Offer him contact details (both in and out of hours) to use if the abuse escalates or if any children are involved.

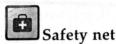

Further reading

1. NICE guidance (2016) *Domestic violence and abuse*. [Online]. Available at: www.nice.org.uk/guidance/qs116 [Accessed 5 February 2017].

2. National Violence Helpline. [Online]. Available at: www.nationaldomesticviolencehelpline.org.uk [Accessed 5 February 2017].

3. Women's Aid. [Online]. Available at: www.womensaid.org.uk [Accessed 5 February 2017].

4. Mankind Initiative. [Online]. Available at: http://new.mankind.org.uk [Accessed 5 February 2017].

5. Men's Advice Line. [Online]. Available at: www.mensadviceline.org.uk [Accessed 5 February 2017].

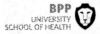

30. Erectile dysfunction

Instructions to candidates

Name:	Derek Kelly
Age:	62 years old
Past medical history:	Hypertension
Medication:	Ramipril 2.5 mg od
Social history:	Works as accountant
	Lives with wife

Instructions to patients

Opening statement

It's a bit embarrassing, but I hope you may be able to help.

Background

- You are a 62-year-old accountant.

- You live at home with your wife. You have 2 children aged 30 and 28 who no longer live at home.

- For the last two years, you have been struggling to have sexual intercourse with your wife as you cannot maintain an erection.

- You are embarrassed to discuss this and did not want to come today. Your wife made the appointment.

- It is putting a strain on your relationship. Initially, your wife accepted that it is 'part of getting older', but as time has gone on, it has been increasingly upsetting and frustrating for both of you.

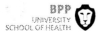

30. Erectile dysfunction

- You have no concerns at home, and feel that you have a healthy relationship with your wife. You are worried that she is upset as you used to have a 'very healthy' sex life.

- If asked, you were under stress two years ago when you had difficulties at work with your boss putting excessive demands on you. This has been resolved, but you think this may have been a trigger for your symptoms and you now worry about maintaining an erection, which is making it worse.

- If asked, you think that this is related to stress and worry. You came today for reassurance that you are still healthy and would like to discuss getting a prescription for Viagra®.

- If asked about your mood, you feel much more able to manage things now; your mood is stable. If asked, your energy levels, sleep and appetite are normal.

- You still have morning erections, and are able to maintain masturbatory erections. You have no problems with ejaculation.

- If asked, your libido is normal, you have no loss of secondary sexual characteristics (no loss of pubic or facial hair).

- If asked, you have no prostatic symptoms (no urgency/frequency/nocturia, poor stream/post-micturition dribble).

- You are well in yourself and have no systemic symptoms/weight loss.

- You take ramipril for hypertension, which you were diagnosed with ten years ago. You are compliant with your medication.

- You take no other medication, including over the counter medications or illicit substances.

- You have no other medical or surgical history.

- You have never smoked. You drink one bottle of wine per week.

- If asked, you play golf twice weekly and enjoy this.

BPP
UNIVERSITY
SCHOOL OF HEALTH

- You would like to be prescribed medication to help you get and maintain an erection. If the doctor agrees to prescribe this today, or after investigations, you will be satisfied. However, if the doctor refuses to prescribe this, you will continue to question why and leave unsatisfied.

- You would be agreeable to having further investigations, including blood tests.

- You would not like to have any intimate examinations today, but would be happy to return for this. You agree to any other examinations today.

Data gathering, technical and assessment skills

History

- Establish how long has this been going on for.

- Ask about any triggers that he might be able to identify.

- What prompted him to consult today? Has anything changed recently?

- It is important to ask about masturbatory and early morning erections – if these are maintained, it suggests a psychological cause, and you can reassure him that everything physically is working.

- Ask about previous erections – has he ever had a problem before?

- Does he have any problems with ejaculation or orgasm?

- What impact is this having on his relationship?

- Enquire about his sexual relationship – is he in a heterosexual or homosexual relationship? Is your partner male or female? How is it affecting the relationship?

- Does he have any other medical conditions? (You may want to ask specifically about some medical conditions – such as diabetes or previous urological surgery (eg vasectomy).)

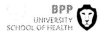

- Ask about risk factors – does he smoke? How much alcohol does he drink? Does he take any illicit substances?

- Has he tried anything to try to manage this already?

- Does he have any prostatic symptoms? – nocturia/frequency of micturition/poor stream/post-micturition dribble.

Examination

- Erectile dysfunction can be an early marker of cardiovascular disease (CVD), so a cardiovascular examination is required – check peripheral pulses, blood pressure, waist circumference and body mass index (BMI).

- Male genital examination – assess testicular size and body hair (if reduced, may suggest hypogonadism), examine the penis for anatomical deformity (eg Peyronie's disease, phimosis).

- Prostate examination in patients with lower urinary tract symptoms and men over the age of 50.

- It is unlikely you will be expected in the exam to carry out the full examination, but it is important that you can explain to the patient what examination you would like to carry out – and why.

Examination findings:

- BP 132/86
- BMI 22.3
- Waist circumference – normal
- Genital and prostate examination declined today

Interpersonal skills

- It is important to have practised and be familiar with asking questions relating to sexual health, as it is important to look comfortable when asking personal questions; the patient may feel anxious or be embarrassed, as in this case.

- Establish the reason for him presenting at this stage; why has he consulted now and not before?

Ideas, concerns, expectations

- Does he have any thoughts about any underlying cause? 'You mentioned that this started when you were under stress...' This feedback will show the examiner you are actively listening and may prompt his ideas to be revealed.

- Find out what impact this is having on his life and his relationship. Is this his main worry? 'You said that your wife asked you to attend today; how is this affecting you and your relationship?'

- Did he have any thoughts on how this could be managed?

- In cases where there is a third party, it can be useful to establish what his wife's ideas, concerns and expectations are as well.

Clinical management

- The underlying cause needs to be established, as erectile dysfunction is a symptom and not a diagnosis. Here, it seems to be psychological in origin.

- Other causes of erectile dysfunction include (this list is not exhaustive):

  - Vascular – hypertension, diabetes, smoking, generalised CVD

  - Endocrine – hypogonadism, hyperprolactinaemia, thyroid disease

  - Neurological – diabetes, spinal cord trauma, Parkinson's disease

  - Surgical – previous pelvic surgery, prostate surgery

  - Anatomical – penile curvature, Peyronie's disease

  - Medication – both prescribed and non-prescribed (eg antihypertensives, antidepressants, marijuana, beta blockers)

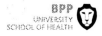

- Psychological – depression, stress, relationship difficulties, performance anxiety

- This list may seem overwhelming, but it will usually become apparent what the underlying cause is. However, it is worth acknowledging early in the consultation that you might not be able to fully manage this in one consultation – they will need to return for examination, bloods etc.

- Erectile dysfunction can be an early marker of CVD or a symptom of established CVD so it is important to carry out a cardiovascular assessment on examination and with blood tests.

- It is important to rule out other causes with blood tests:
  - Early morning testosterone to check for hypogonadism
  - Prostate specific antigen (PSA) if the history suggests
  - Lipids and fasting glucose to check cardiovascular risk
  - TFTs if suggested by history

- Make a **shared management plan** with the patient:
  - Discuss lifestyle changes – stopping smoking, reducing alcohol intake, stopping illicit drug use, lose weight.

  - Offer PDE-5 inhibitor (provided there are no contraindications) to all patients, regardless of cause and can be offered whilst awaiting investigation.

  - Discuss relationship issues – does he feel he needs any extra support here? You could signpost to relationship counselling services.

- This is a good opportunity to demonstrate a shared management plan:
  - 'There are things that we can do to help and things you can do; now that I've told you more about some of the causes of erectile problems (smoking, alcohol, etc), is there anything you think you might be able to do?'

- 'We can manage this with lifestyle changes as well as medication; did you have any ideas about where you would like to start?'

- Referral criteria:

  - Hypogonadism (low serum testosterone, clinical features) – refer to endocrinology

  - Cannot use PDE-5 inhibitors – either a contraindication or not effective

  - Previous trauma (penile or spinal injury) or anatomical abnormality of the penis

Safety net

- Offer a review appointment to follow up on blood tests and complete the physical examination.

- If you have started treatment you could review effectiveness at the follow-up.

- If you have started Sildenafil it is important to inform the patient to attend Accident and Emergency if he has an erection lasting more than four hours (priapism).

Further reading

NICE CKS (2014) *Erectile dysfunction*. [Online]. Available at: https://cks.nice.org.uk/erectile-dysfunction [Accessed 5 February 2017].

31. Asthma

Instructions to candidates

Name:	Anna Simpson
Age:	33 years old
Past medical history:	Asthma
	Hypothyroidism
Medication:	Levothyroxine 100 micrograms OD
	Salbutamol 2 puffs BD
	Seretide 500 1 puff BD
Social history:	Lives with 5-year-old daughter
	Smokes 20/day
	Works as a cleaner
Last consultation 2 months ago:	DNA asthma review following asthma exacerbation
Best PEFR:	450 L/min

Instructions to patients

Opening statement

> *I've got a chest infection, I think I need antibiotics.*

Background

- You are a 33-year-old cleaner.

- You have a past medical history of asthma and 'low thyroid'.

- You take 'a couple of puffers' and your thyroid tablets. You do not take any over the counter medications regularly.

- You state that your asthma is well controlled but over the last two days you have been coughing more and using your blue inhaler more.

- Your chest feels tighter than normal over the last two days. You have been using two puffs of your blue inhaler five times a day.

- If asked, this will relieve the tightness in your chest for about two hours.

- You have not been feeling feverish.

- You have a dry cough, with no green or blood stained sputum.

- There is no history of recent travel.

- If asked, you have never been into hospital with your asthma.

- You have had 2 exacerbations of your asthma in the last 12 months, requiring steroid courses on each occasion. The last exacerbation was 2 months ago.

- If asked about your asthma control, you state that it is well controlled.

- If the doctor explores this more, you state that you use your blue inhaler twice a day normally.

- If asked about night-time symptoms, you state that you wake up needing your blue inhaler a couple of times a month.

- You smoke 20 cigarettes a day.

- If asked about smoking, you state that you are aware you need to stop, but would like some support in doing so. If the doctor signposts you towards this support you accept it.

- You are worried that you have needed two courses of steroids in the last year and think that to prevent you having further exacerbations of your asthma you need antibiotics on this occasion.

- If the doctor asks you why you failed to attend your follow-up appointment after your last exacerbation you state that you didn't think you needed to be seen as you felt better.

- If the doctor doesn't clearly explain the rationale for not prescribing antibiotics you will not be satisfied with the consultation.

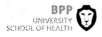

- If the doctor explains that no antibiotics are needed, and gives a clear explanation, you accept this.

- If the doctor suggests that your asthma is not as well controlled as you thought, you will be surprised. If they explain it clearly and sensitively you will agree that your asthma control could be improved as you are bothered by it most days. If this is explained well, you agree to attend a follow-up appointment, now that you understand why it is important.

Data gathering, technical and assessment skills

History

- Ask about why she thinks she has a chest infection – what symptoms is she experiencing?

- How long has she had these symptoms for?

- Ask about symptoms of a chest infection – fever? Cough? Purulent sputum?

- Any symptoms that may suggest another cause – haemoptysis? Chest pain?

- Assess whether this is likely to be an asthma exacerbation – how frequently has she been using her reliever inhaler? Does this relieve her symptoms? For how long?

- She mentioned that her asthma is well controlled normally – what does this mean to her? How often does her asthma cause her symptoms? How often does she use her reliever inhaler?

  Note. It is important to enquire more about what she means by 'good control'. Patients may think their asthma is well controlled, but on further questioning this lady's asthma is quite poorly controlled, as she needs to use her inhaler daily and is having frequent exacerbations.

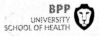

- It might also be useful to check her understanding of what her inhalers are for. Does she understand about preventer and reliever inhalers and how they should be used?

- To learn more about her asthma control ask about: any previous hospital admissions? ITU admissions? This may suggest brittle asthma.

- How frequently is she having exacerbations?

- Enquire about why she failed to attend her follow-up appointment.

- Is she a smoker? This is a good opportunity for health promotion.

Examination
- Whilst taking the history assess for work of breathing and respiratory distress: is the patient able to complete their sentences, are they using accessory muscles? Are they visibly cyanosed?

- Check pulse rate, respiratory rate, oxygen saturations, blood pressure and peak flow – to assess the severity of the exacerbation of asthma. **Note.** Peak flow, oxygen saturations, RR and pulse rate should be included in all asthma exacerbation consultations.

- Temperature if symptoms of infection.

- Chest examination – assessing air entry, and listening for signs of consolidation or wheeze.

Findings:

- No respiratory distress, talking clearly in full sentences
- No visible cyanosis, O_2 saturations 95% in air
- Pulse rate 96, respiratory rate 20, BP 110/75
- PEFR: 300 L/min

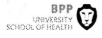

Interpersonal skills

Ideas, concerns, expectations

- She has clearly stated that she thinks she may have a chest infection, but check back with her to confirm this is her interpretation of what is going on, and find out why she thinks she has a chest infection.

- Is there anything that was worrying her about this?

- What impact is this having on her life?

- She mentioned that she would like antibiotics – find out why she felt this was needed. Was there anything else that she was hoping for today?

Clinical management

- This case opens up more issues than just the case of managing the acute exacerbation of asthma, and the examiner will be looking for your ability to identify and manage these.

- These issues include:

  1. Management of the acute exacerbation of asthma

  2. Smoking cessation – an opportunity for health promotion

  3. Understanding of longer-term asthma control, including issues with compliance

- From the history and examination findings, this is a moderate acute exacerbation of asthma:

  - PEFR > 50% of predicted

  - No features of severe asthma (PEFR 33–50%, HR > 110, inability to complete sentences)

- This is managed with the following:

  1. Prednisolone 40–50 mg daily for 5 days

2. Inhaled β2 agonist (salbutamol) via a spacer – advise the patient to use up to 10 puffs (start with 4 puffs, and increase in increments of 2 puffs) 4 times a day

3. Safety net to seek medical attention if:

   i) Needing salbutamol more than four hourly
   ii) PEFR worsens
   iii) Symptoms worsen – feeling more short of breath/unwell

4. Follow up within one week

- It was also identified in the history that this patient is expecting antibiotics. There are no signs of an infective process (no temperature, purulent sputum, or chest signs) so antibiotics would not be indicated here. You will need to explain this to the patient. There are useful leaflets that you can give to the patient supporting this, such as: http://patient.info/health/chest-infection.

- One of the issues in this case is a poor understanding of her asthma control. Patients may often say that their asthma control is good, but it is important to check what they mean by this and ask three important questions:

   1. How often does asthma limit your activities?
   2. How often does asthma cause you symptoms at night?
   3. How often does asthma limit exercise?

- Asthma control can also be assessed by how often they are using their reliever inhaler – she is using hers daily which suggests poor control and/or lack of understanding of how her inhalers should be used.

- Use this opportunity to address this – it is unlikely you will be able to fully address this in the consultation, but you can highlight that she needs to have an asthma review to check her inhaler technique, check her understanding of what her inhalers do and give her a written action plan for what to do when her breathing deteriorates.

- **Note.** It is part of the NICE guidelines and BTS guidelines that all patients with asthma should be given a written action plan so it would be a good idea here to address this.

- It is also useful to address the topic of smoking cessation, which again you may not be able to cover in this consultation, but you can point out that this is something that she might like to consider and advise her that you can offer support for this.

 Safety net

- It is important that all patients should be followed up after an asthma exacerbation – advise this patient to book in for an asthma review in one week.

- Advise them that if their breathing deteriorates (more short of breath, difficulty breathing, or if needing salbutamol > 10 puffs every 4 hours) they should be reviewed straight away.

 Further reading

1. BTS/SIGN (2016) *Management of asthma*. [Online]. Available at: www.brit-thoracic.org.uk/document-library/clinical-information/asthma/btssign-asthma-guideline-2016/ [Accessed 11 February 2017].

2. BTS (2009) *Management of community acquired pneumonia in adults*. [Online]. Available at: www.brit-thoracic.org.uk/document-library/clinical-information/pneumonia/adult-pneumonia/a-quick-reference-guide-bts-guidelines-for-the-management-of-community-acquired-pneumonia-in-adults/ [Accessed 11 February 2017].

3. NICE CKS (2016) *Asthma*. [Online]. Available at: https://cks.nice.org.uk/asthma [Accessed 11 February 2017].

32. Nocturnal enuresis

Instructions to candidates

Name:	Asim Khan
Age:	6 years old
Past medical history:	Nil
Medication:	Nil regular
Immunisations:	Up to date

Instructions to patients

Opening statement

Hello doctor, I'm a bit worried about my son's bed wetting.

Background

- You are Talia Khan, Asim's mother. You have not brought Asim with you today as he is at school.

- You are concerned that Asim has never been dry at night.

- You have a daughter aged ten and also your husband at home.

- Asim will usually wet the bed once or twice a week.

- It happens once a night, and is quite a large amount. If asked, it seems to be a few hours after going to bed.

- You know that it isn't his fault, but you do find it very frustrating and sometimes this shows to Asim. You are never physically violent, if asked, you just 'huff and puff a bit' whilst changing the sheets and he can see that you are annoyed.

- If asked, you do not punish Asim for bedwetting.

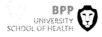

32. Nocturnal enuresis

- Asim is now starting to become upset by this as he is getting tired the following day. This doesn't affect your husband and daughter at the moment, as they sleep through the noise.

- He is dry by day and has been since he was two and a half years old.

- He is at school at the moment but is a happy child and there are no concerns at school.

- There are no issues at home. Your relationship with your husband is fine and there have been no major stressors/life events recently.

- Asim has his own bedroom and easy access to the bathroom which is next door.

- You are concerned as your daughter was dry at night by the age of four years old, and are worried that there is something wrong with Asim.

- If asked, so far you have tried limiting Asim's fluid intake in the evening and done a star chart for the days he doesn't wet the bed, but you haven't noticed any improvement, so you abandoned both ideas after two weeks.

- He was born at term, and has no medical problems, including no history of urine infections.

- If asked, you think that Asim drinks a normal amount of fluids at home, but will have fizzy drinks in the evening.

- He opens his bowels regularly on a daily basis, and you have not noticed that he is constipated or straining.

- If asked, you don't know what could be wrong, but you came today for some guidance on how you could manage this. You wonder if some medication may be helpful.

- If the doctor dismisses your concerns, or doesn't explain things to you clearly you become demanding for medication.

- If the doctor explores different options with you and involves you in the management plan, you would like to try an enuresis alarm in the first instance.

- You are wary of trying star charts again, as they failed to work previously, but if the doctor sensitively advises that they may take a while to work, you would be willing to give it another try.

- If the doctor suggest a 'wait and see approach' you are reluctant for this, and would rather some intervention, as you and Asim are finding it quite tiresome.

Data gathering, technical and assessment skills

History

- Ask more about his bed wetting – it can be helpful to start with an open question, such as 'Can you tell me more about his bed wetting?' as you will often obtain a lot of useful information, and can then ask more direct and specific questions – this is a useful consultation technique that can be applied to most scenarios.

- Has he ever been dry by night? If so, how long for?

- Is he dry by day? At what age was this achieved?

- How often is he wetting the bed?

- Does it appear to be at a particular time of night?

- Is he waking after bed wetting?

- Find out what she does and how she reacts when she find the bed wet. Does she involve Asim in changing the bed sheets?

- What has she tried to manage this already? How long did she try these for? How successful were they?

- What is his fluid intake like during the day?

- What are his bowel habits like? Is he prone to constipation? (Constipation can make enuresis worse.)

- Enquire about home and school circumstances – is there anything going on at home or at school that you think might be worrying him?

- Does he have easy access to the toilet at night?

Examination

- Urinalysis is indicated if the child is unwell, has symptoms of UTI or diabetes mellitus or if they have previously been dry at night and the onset is recent (suspected UTI).

- General examination – check height and weight if any suggestion of maltreatment or general ill health.

- Examination of abdomen – to assess for constipation if history suggests, palpable bladder (which may suggest neurological cause).

- Examination of spine and lower limb neurology if suspecting neurological cause (eg spina bifida).

Interpersonal skills

Ideas, concerns, expectations

- Does she and/or Asim have any thoughts about why he is not dry by night?

- Pick up on the cue that she is finding it frustrating and explore what she finds frustrating – 'You mentioned that you can find it quite frustrating; is there anything in particular that worries you about this?'

- Find out if there are any ways she would like you to help, or if she had any expectations of how this might be managed – 'You mentioned that you have tried a few measures, was there anything you were hoping I might be able to suggest or help you with today?'

- It would also be useful to establish the impact this is having on the family and empathise with the patient – 'This problem can be very frustrating for parents and you are obviously worried about this. How is this affecting you and the rest of your family? Does Asim think there is a problem?'

Clinical management

- Reassure the mother that as Asim is wetting the bed once or twice a week it is likely that this will settle with time, and the vast majority of children, given time, will stop bed wetting.

- Explain the reason that children wet the bed – 'Asim's bladder isn't telling his brain that it is full, so he doesn't know that he needs to wake up to empty his bladder.'

- You could explain that the aim of management is to allow the brain to learn that the bladder is full at night so that he knows to wake up and go to the toilet.

- Discuss management options which could include active intervention or a watchful waiting approach to give things time to settle spontaneously – discuss and offer these options to the parents to share the management.

- Reassure the mother that as Asim's bladder capacity increases, and as he learns to wake to the sensation of a full bladder, this may settle with a 'wait and see' approach.

- This is where establishing the parents' and the patient's expectations are important as management will depend on the impact on family life and whether they are looking for active management or reassurance, as well as whether they are looking for intervention for a short-term gain or a longer-term management strategy.

- Direct the patient towards self-help websites – ERIC is an organisation that provides information for parents and children which can be useful.

- If active management is required, discuss with the mother that there are different approaches, and she can adopt all or none of them:

  - Do not restrict fluid intake. This is important to help develop bladder capacity, and allow Asim's bladder to get used to the normal sensation of being full and emptying. You could suggest a star chart system for Asim for the days where he drinks adequate fluids.

  - Avoid caffeine and fizzy drinks (they can have an irritant effect on the bladder).

  - Encourage regular toileting during the day – this will help to develop bladder capacity and a recognition of the feeling of bladder fullness.

  - Encourage Asim to go to the toilet before bed. You could suggest a reward system for this also.

  - Avoid waking or lifting – this doesn't allow Asim to get used to the sensation of bladder fullness and a recognition to wake up in response to this.

  - Encourage Asim to get involved in changing the bed, so that he feels involved in his management.

- You could also discuss treatment with an enuresis alarm – this is an alarm that should wake the child when wetness in the bed is detected. The child should then be encouraged to get up and go to the toilet to finish passing urine. In time, Asim would then learn to recognise that his bladder is full prior to the alarm sounding. This may take weeks or months to take effect, and should be used in combination with reward systems.

- This case is a good opportunity to demonstrate that you can take a shared management approach: you can discuss the options of watchful waiting, reward systems and lifestyle changes and enuresis alarms for this case. By giving the mother the information, you can reach a shared decision for the best management for Asim.

Safety net

- Explain that these management options will not work immediately; that they may have progress then relapses. You could offer follow-up in a few weeks' time to monitor progress, and see how the family are managing with the changes.

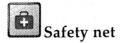 **Further reading**

Eric, the Children's Bowel & Bladder Charity. [Online]. Available at: www.eric.org.uk [Accessed 11 February 2017].

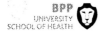

33. Obesity

Instructions to candidates

Name:	Francesca Holden
Age:	40 years old
Past medical history:	Non-ulcer dyspepsia
Medication:	Omeprazole 20 mg prn

Instructions to patients

Opening statement

> *I'd like you to help me with my weight.*

Background

- You are a 40-year-old office worker.

- You are married and have a 10-year-old daughter.

- You have struggled with your weight most of your adult life, but since you had your daughter you feel that your weight has become more of a problem.

- Your father died three months ago – he suffered a heart attack and had diabetes and this made you realise that your weight puts you at risk of developing these conditions as well.

- You have acid reflux, which is controlled with omeprazole when required.

- You do notice the reflux is worse when you have a fatty meal.

- You have no other medical problems.

- You have previously tried meal replacement drinks but found these too restrictive.

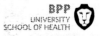

- You do not smoke.

- You drink one bottle of wine per week.

- If asked, you eat porridge for breakfast and a healthy meal at dinner time with the family. You think that your lunch and snacks could be healthier. You often eat at the work canteen for lunch and would usually have the main meal and dessert. You would then snack on chocolate or crisps in the afternoon at your desk.

- You heard from your friend that there is a tablet that you can take to help with weight loss and you would like this to be prescribed today.

- You are expecting the doctor to tell you that you are overweight.

- If the doctor tells you that your weight is categorised as 'obese' and verging on 'morbidly obese', you are quite shocked and upset that you have 'let yourself go' this much.

- This also upsets you as you want to teach your daughter healthy eating habits and want to 'lead by example'.

- If the doctor discusses changes to your diet, you are aware that you snack quite a lot in the afternoon, and think that swapping these snacks for fruit would be a good place to start.

- You also would like to start playing tennis again, which you used to enjoy, and if the doctor discusses exercise with you, you agree you will start this up again once a week initially.

- If the doctor discusses structured weight management services, you think this may be difficult to work into your lifestyle, so would like to make dietary changes to begin with.

- You were expecting to leave with a prescription for medication today, and will be quite dissatisfied if the doctor does not prescribe medication. If, however, they give you a reasonable explanation of why they are not prescribing the medication today you accept this.

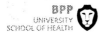

- If the doctor agrees to prescribe medication you will accept a prescription.

Data gathering, technical and assessment skills

History

- Find out more about why she wants help with her weight.

- Find out more about why has she consulted about this now. Has there been a trigger for why she feels she needs help with her weight now?

- Ask about what she has tried already to lose weight.

- Does she have any other medical conditions?

- How much exercise does she do each week?

- Ask about smoking and alcohol – a good opportunity for health promotion.

- Find out more about her diet – 'Could you explain to me what you might eat in an average day?' How often does she eat takeaway? How often does she eat sugary/processed foods?

- Is there anywhere you think you might be able to make changes in her diet or lifestyle?

Examination
- Weight: 90 kg

- Height: 1.65 m

- BMI: 33.1

- It might also be useful to check waist circumference and blood pressure

---

Interpersonal skills

Ideas, concerns, expectations

- This would be a good case to start with an open statement or question, as she is likely to give you answers to a lot of questions you may have. 'Tell me a bit more about that...', for example.

- What does she think about being classed as obese? 'Your weight is showing that you are classified in the obese category, does this come as a surprise to you?' or 'How does this make you feel?'

- Has anything happened that worried her and made her consult now?

- Why does she want to lose weight? Has anything happened that has triggered her consultation now?

- What worries her about her weight? What does she think might be the challenges to her losing weight?

- 'You mentioned you would like me to help you, was there anything in particular you had in mind?'

Clinical management

- This should be a multi-faceted approach, incorporating education about diet and exercise, and offering or discussing psychological therapies and medication.

- You could also discuss with her the implications of an unhealthy weight. It sounds like she already has some understanding after her father's ill health, but this could be an opportunity for health education.

- It might be useful to explore what this lady's diet is like normally, by asking her to keep a food diary. You can then educate her on a healthy diet and ask her where she thinks she may be able to make changes to her diet and lifestyle, giving her the opportunity to control her own health.

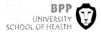

33. Obesity

- Options for management should be discussed and allow the patient to reach a decision. These options include:
  - Diet and exercise advice with regular weighing and support in practice (eg with practice nurse)
  - Referral to structured weight management services
  - Commence Orlistat
  - Referral for bariatric surgery
- Dietary advice should recommend a nutritionally balanced diet that is sustainable in the long term. Severely calorie restricted diets are not recommended unless under specialist supervision.
  - At least five portions of fruit and vegetables per day
  - Lower fat meat, poultry and dairy
  - Starchy foods – brown varieties if possible, eg brown rice, wholemeal bread
  - Cut out fizzy, sugary drinks and alcohol
  - Cut back on foods high in fat and sugar
  - Reduce salt intake to no more than 6 g/day
  - Use low fat cooking methods eg boiling, grilling rather than frying
- Combined with exercise – 30 minutes 5 times a week. Explain this doesn't have to be intense exercise, but has to be enough to raise the heart rate and start to break a slight sweat.
- You could offer written advice on a healthy balanced diet and exercise. A good leaflet is the 'Your weight your health' leaflet from the NHS: www.htmc.co.uk/resource/data/htmc1/docs/How%20to%20take%20control%20of%20your%20weight.pdf.

- This patient is a candidate for Orlistat. This reduces fat absorption and should be iterated that it should be combined with dietary changes:
  - Can be prescribed to patients with a BMI > 30
  - Or a BMI > 28 kg/m² with significant comorbidities
  - Prescribe for 3 months and re-weigh. Only continue if weight loss of > 5%
  - Advise of side effects which include abdominal cramps, fatty stools, anal leakage and faecal urgency, and are significantly worse if non-compliant with low fat diet
  - Also advise that impairment of fat soluble vitamins (A, D, E and K) is impaired, so a healthy balanced diet is important

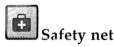**Safety net**

- Offer follow-up to re-weigh; you could suggest they bring a food and exercise diary too.
- Aim for weight loss no more than 1 kg/week.

Further reading

1. NICE CKS (2015) *Obesity*. [Online]. Available at: https://cks.nice.org.uk/obesity#!topicsummary [Accessed 11 February 2017].
2. NHS Choices. *Obesity*. [Online]. Available at: www.nhs.uk/conditions/obesity/Pages/Introduction.aspx [Accessed 11 February 2017].

34. Peripheral arterial disease

Instructions to candidates

Name:	Alan Mansey
Age:	57 years old
Past medical history:	Hypertension
Occupation:	Security guard
Social history:	Smoker 30/day
	Alcohol 14 units/week
	Lives alone

Instructions to patients

Opening statement

> *I've been getting cramps in my leg.*

Background

- You are a 57-year-old security guard in a shopping centre.

- You live alone following your divorce three years ago.

- You have two grown-up children.

- You have been getting pains in the back of your left calf for about six months now, but it is progressively getting worse and affecting your work.

- You describe the pain as a cramp.

- The pain is worse when you are walking and, if asked, it settles a few seconds after stopping.

- You haven't noticed any relation to your posture. If asked, you do not find the pain is any better if you are standing up or leaning forwards.

BPP
UNIVERSITY
SCHOOL OF HEALTH

- The pain will usually occur after walking to the end of your road, which you think is a couple of hundred yards. It also occurs at work, after walking one length of the shopping centre.

- You are worried that you may not be able to run after someone at work, and worry that people may say that you aren't able to do your job properly.

- You have no associated symptoms of tingling or numbness in the legs. You have no back pain.

- If asked, you have had no night pain or rest pain.

- If asked, you have not noticed any changes to the colour of your skin, and you have not noticed any broken skin or wounds.

- You have smoked since you were 17. You smoke 30 cigarettes a day since your divorce 3 years ago.

- You were told that your blood pressure was high at a routine check-up two years ago but didn't want to start taking any tablets.

- You have no other medical conditions.

- You are worried this could be a blood clot, as you are aware that this can cause cramp in the calf.

- If the doctor gives you a diagnosis of claudication, you are not surprised that it is due to your circulation, and are glad to have a diagnosis.

- You are not keen on taking tablets and would resist this if the doctor suggests you start medication.

- If, however, they explain clearly the rationale for prescribing medication, you agree to consider this and would like some information to read before you make your decision.

- You would agree to a referral to a structured exercise programme.

- If the doctor discusses management of risk factors, including stopping smoking, you agree to this. You decline referral to a stop smoking clinic as you feel that you have enough incentive to stop.

Data gathering, technical and assessment skills

History

- Ask more about the pain:

  - How long has he had the cramps for?

  - Where are the cramps? Is it confined to one leg or is it bilateral?

  - When does he get the pain? What makes the pain worse? Does anything make the pain better?

  - Does he have any other symptoms with this – ask specifically about tingling, numbness and weakness.

- Ask about red flags:

  - Has he had any night pain?
  - Any rest pain?
  - Has he noticed any changes to the colour of his feet/toes?
  - Has he noticed any broken skin (suggesting ulcers)?

- Identify risk factors:

  - Does he smoke? If not, has he ever smoked? How long has he smoked for and how many cigarettes?

  - Other relevant medical history – high cholesterol? High blood pressure? Previous heart disease? Diabetes?

- Rule out important differentials:

  - Neurogenic claudication – pain relieved by leaning forwards

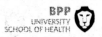

- DVT – suggested if acute pain and swelling
- Arthritis – joints more affected
- You could also consider biochemical causes – myopathy, vitamin D deficiency

Interpersonal skills

Ideas, concerns, expectations

- Enquire about what he thinks might be causing his symptoms – does he have any ideas what might be going on?

- What prompted him to consult now? It has been troubling him for six months; has anything changed recently?

- It is important to pick up on the cue that he gave about it affecting his work – how is it affecting him at work? What impact has this had? Is this his main concern, or is there anything else that worries him about this?

- Does he have any thoughts or expectations about how this may be managed, or how you may be able to help him with these symptoms?

Red flags
- Night pain
- Rest pain
- On examination:
  - Pale
  - Pulseless
  - Perishingly cold
  - Paraesthesia
  - Pain
  - Paralysis

These suggest critical or acute limb ischaemia and need urgent or same day review by Vascular team.

Examination

- Examine both legs checking for peripheral pulses

- Examine the feet checking colour, sensation, skin changes, broken skin or evidence of ulceration

- Check for risk factors for vascular disease – BP, waist circumference, BMI

Findings:

- Leg pulses intact
- No skin changes/ulceration
- BP 134/89
- BMI 23.5
- Waist circumference – normal

Clinical management

- It is important here to rule out an acute limb ischaemia that would warrant immediate referral to hospital, or critical limb ischaemia that would need urgent referral (this is usually best achieved by speaking to the vascular surgery on-call team).

  - Acute limb ischaemia – 6 Ps – Pale, Pulseless, Perishingly cold, Paraesthesia, Pain, Paralysis. May be acute (due to embolus) or insidious onset (due to thrombus, which is typically preceded by a history of claudication).

  - Critical limb ischaemia – rest and night pain, dependent redness, absent pulses.

- This is a case of intermittent claudication – he has no night or rest symptoms and examination is normal with intact pulses and no features of critical or acute limb ischaemia.

- It is important to explain this diagnosis to the patient without using jargon, and check their understanding.

- There are a few components to management here:

  - Advice regarding stopping smoking – explain to the patient that smoking damages the blood vessels

- Advice on graded exercise or referral to a structured exercise programme

- Management of other cardiovascular risk factors – optimising blood pressure control, checking cholesterol and managing this, starting an antiplatelet

- This is another example of where you can share the management – you can discuss the different components of management, and prioritise which you will target first by making the plan with the patient.

- You could explain that if these conservative measures fail you can consider prescribing naftidrofuryl oxalate, which is a vasodilator.

Safety net

- You could give this patient a leaflet on peripheral arterial disease.
  Note. Whenever giving a patient a leaflet you need to explain why you are giving this, and what information they can expect the leaflet to cover. This will show the examiner that you understand what a leaflet is for; simply giving out a leaflet may not demonstrate you have 'ticked this box' to the examiner.

- Advise the patient to seek immediate medical attention if he has a pale, cold or numb, weak or acutely painful leg or foot.

- He needs to seek review if he is experiencing rest pain or ulceration, which suggests critical limb ischaemia.

Further reading

NICE (2012) *Peripheral Arterial Disease: diagnosis and management*. [Online]. Available at: www.nice.org.uk/guidance/CG147 [Accessed 11 February 2017].

35. Giant cell arteritis

Instructions to candidates

Name:	Jean Thompson
Age:	75 years old
Past medical history:	Diverticulosis
	Hysterectomy
Occupation:	Retired seamstress
Social history:	Ex-smoker (20 years ago)
	Alcohol 6 units/week

Instructions to patients

Opening statement

I think I've got a migraine doctor.

Background

- You are a 75-year-old retired seamstress.

- You live with your husband who has Parkinson's disease.

- You were diagnosed with diverticulosis 3 years ago, but have had no problems related to this recently. You also had a hysterectomy 20 years ago.

- You smoked until 20 years ago. You drink 6 units of alcohol each week.

- Over the last 3 days you have had a headache.

- If asked, you do not drive.

- You've been feeling a bit run down for the last week with generalised aching and fatigue.

- Only answer if asked specifically:
  - Location: right-sided headache
  - Nature: it is a sharp, constant pain
  - Precipitating factors: you have avoided eating as this makes the pain unbearable
  - Visual problems: your vision has been a 'bit funny' since yesterday. If explored further, you state that it is like someone is holding a curtain across your eye. It is on the right side of your right eye. You have no pain in your eye. You have no double vision or flashing lights
  - Vomiting? No
  - Associated symptoms: you have been feeling tired and had aching in your shoulders a couple of days ago
  - Is the headache worse on lying or standing? It's not worse on lying or standing
  - Any preceding head injury? No
  - How quickly did the pain develop? It developed slowly over the last three days
- You think this may be a migraine as you called your daughter and she said that she gets migraines with visual problems.
- You would like some of the 'migraine pills' that you daughter is given.
- If the doctor suggests this is not a migraine, you are quite surprised as your daughter told you she gets similar symptoms.
- If they agree it is a migraine, you ask for some migraine tablets and will be happy with a prescription issued.
- If the doctor explains clearly this may be a more serious condition, you accept any medication they may suggest. If they are not clear, or dismiss your idea that this could be a migraine, you keep asking for 'migraine tablets' and do not allow the consultation to move forward.

- If the doctor tells you that you need to go to hospital, you refuse. You state that you are waiting for a delivery at home, and your husband would not be able to manage this on his own.

- Even if the doctor tells you that this could lead to permanent visual loss, which can affect the other eye, you refuse to go to hospital. You understand the risks and are able to relay this back to the doctor, if asked. You state that you cannot leave your husband at home to take a delivery on his own. You will go to hospital tomorrow if that's what is needed.

- You accept any medication that may be needed and agree to go to hospital tomorrow.

- If the doctor discusses with you about permanent visual loss, you are quite scared by this thought, but state 'I'll face that bridge when I come to it'.

- If the doctor discusses with you the need for extra support at home, you decline this at present, but may discuss this with your daughter and husband.

Data gathering, technical and assessment skills

History

- Establish what she means by migraine – what symptoms is she having?

- Ask more about the nature of the headache:

  - Where is the headache felt (unilateral/bilateral/location in head)?

  - What is the nature of the pain? Sharp/stabbing/pressure?

  - Associated symptoms – vomiting? Visual symptoms? – ask specifically about double vision, blurred vision, visual field defects. Neurological symptoms – ask about 'tingling', weakness, numbness.

- If considering temporal arteritis ask specifically about jaw claudication, symptoms of PMR (shoulder or pelvic girdle pain).

- Are the headaches postural?

- Are they worse at any particular time of day?

- Is there any preceding head injury?

- Did the headache develop slowly or was it of sudden onset?

• Does she normally suffer with headaches? Is this different to normal?

• What makes her think that it is a migraine?

• Ask about any previous medical history.

Examination

• Check blood pressure

• Examination of cranial nerves

• Perform full neurological examination if focal neurological symptoms present

• Fundoscopy

• Palpation of temporal arteries

Findings:

• BP 145/85
• Tender over right temporal artery
• Upper limb neurology all normal
• Fundoscopy normal
• Cranial nerves – visual field defect of right temporal area

---

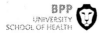

35. Giant cell arteritis

> **Red flags**
>
> - **Suggestive of space occupying lesion:** postural; early morning headache; associated vomiting; focal neurological symptoms; papilloedema on fundoscopy
>
> - **Suggestive of acute pathology, requiring admission:** temporal artery tenderness, jaw claudication, visual symptoms suggestive of GCA; sudden onset to peak intensity suggestive of subarachnoid haemorrhage; associated with fever, neck stiffness, photophobia suggestive of intracranial infection

Interpersonal skills

Ideas, concerns, expectations

- This lady has clearly stated that she thinks she has a migraine – show that you have listened to this: 'You mentioned you think this might be a migraine…' And you could add on 'was there anything else you thought this could be?'

- Establish why she thought this could be a migraine – 'What drew you to this conclusion?'

- How did she feel you might be able to help her today? What was she hoping to leave the consultation with?

- Once you have explained to her the more likely diagnosis of GCA, it is useful to establish if this is something that she has heard of, or what she already understands by this diagnosis.

- Once you have explained the potential long-term complications of GCA, explore how this makes her feel. What are her concerns about this?

Clinical management

- The history here is suggestive of GCA – she is an elderly lady with a new onset unilateral headache with associated jaw claudication, a tender temporal artery on examination and a visual field defect.

BPP
UNIVERSITY
SCHOOL OF HEALTH

- The first priority is to explain this to the patient: 'I suspect you may not have a migraine, but instead have a condition called giant cell arteritis. This is a condition affecting your blood vessels, which can become inflamed and cause a headache. It can affect the blood vessels in your eye, and if not treated can lead to permanent vision problems'.

- This requires an understanding of the referral pathways. If there are visual symptoms then the patient needs urgent (same day) assessment by ophthalmology; if not they need assessment by the medical team. This lady would need to see an ophthalmologist.

- When this lady states that she doesn't want to go to hospital explore her reasons why not.

- If she is refusing, it is important to establish whether she has capacity to make this decision:
  - Can she understand the information?
  - Can she retain the information?
  - Can she weigh up the decision?
  - Can she communicate the decision?

  Remember an unwise decision does not mean that she does not have capacity. And assume she has capacity until you can prove otherwise.

- The issue of her concerned about her husband on his own at home should raise the discussion of whether extra support is required at home; it is unlikely you will cover this during your consultation, but acknowledge this to discuss at the next appointment.

- Given that she has refused referral currently, you need to start management for suspected GCA (given that she has visual symptoms this should be started before waiting for confirmation of diagnosis): Prednisolone 60 mg once daily.

- NICE guidance also recommends commencing her on aspirin 75 mg and a proton-pump inhibitor.

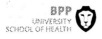

- It would be useful to mention that this is a long-term treatment that will be tapered down slowly over the course of months. Again, this can be prioritised to discuss at a follow-up appointment, but demonstrate that you are aware of this issue. You may want to mention a steroid card, but again this could be dealt with at follow-up.

- Even though she doesn't want to go to hospital today, you could discuss with her whether she would be happy to be referred to the rheumatologist or ophthalmologist to be seen that week. You could discuss with her liaising with these specialists to arrange an assessment the following day.

 Safety net

- You should advise this lady that if she changes her mind, she can still present herself to eye casualty, A&E or return to see you.

- You should arrange to review this lady within 48 hours; hopefully she will have also been reviewed by the rheumatologist and/or ophthalmologist and had a confirmed diagnosis and management plan.

 Further reading

1. NICE CKS (2014) *Giant Cell Arteritis*. [Online]. Available at: https://cks.nice.org.uk/giant-cell-arteritis [Accessed 11 February 2017].

2. European Vasculitis Society. [Online]. Available at: www.vasculitis.org.uk/about-vasculitis/giant-cell-arteritis -temporal-arteritis [Accessed 11 February 2017].

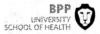

36. A patient with a list

Instructions to candidates

Name:	Sally Findal
Age:	42 years old
Past medical history:	Polycystic ovarian syndrome
	Tennis elbow
Occupation:	Teacher
Social history:	Never smoked
	Alcohol 4 units/week

Instructions to patients

Opening statement

> *Well it's a couple of things today, doctor.*

Background

- You are Sally, a 42-year-old teacher.

- You live at home with your husband and 2 children (aged 11 and 8 years).

- You tell the doctor that you don't come to the doctor's very often, so you've got a few things to discuss today and have written a list.

- If the doctor doesn't ask to see the list you start explaining the problems in the following order, not moving on from each problem until the first is dealt with:

  - Foot pain
  - Stye
  - Blood from back passage

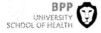

- If the doctor fails to prioritise tasks or establish what the issues are early on in the consultation, you bring up the topic of rectal bleeding in the last minute of the consultation.

- If the doctor asks to see the list and asks which is worrying you the most, you state that the blood from the back passage is what prompted you to book this appointment and you would like to discuss this first.

Foot pain:
- You have had pain in your right foot for about six weeks. It is a pain on the sole of your foot, which is worse when you get out of bed in the morning.

- There is no history of trauma.

- There is not redness or heat around your foot.

- The pain is relieved when you've stretched out your foot or taken a few steps in the morning.

- You've tried paracetamol for pain relief.

- You weren't sure what could be going on; you thought about arthritis or gout.

- It worried you as you think you are too young to suffer from arthritis or gout.

- If the doctor suggests this sounds like plantar fasciitis, you agree to whatever measures they suggest (oral or topical pain killers, steroid injection or referral for surgery).

Stye:
- You noticed a lump on the left upper eyelid a few weeks ago. It appears to have completely settled now but you thought you should still discuss it.

- You had no visual disturbance. There was no pain in your eye.

- As it is settled you are happy if the doctor simply reassures you and advises you to consult if it flares up again and causes any redness or visual disturbance or concerns.

Rectal bleeding:
- Last week on two occasions, you had fresh red blood when wiping after going to the toilet to open your bowels. It was a very small amount, a smear on the toilet paper.

- It last occurred five days ago and you have had no problems since.

- You have never had rectal bleeding before.

- You also noticed that it was 'like passing razor blades' when you opened your bowels.

- There is no blood mixed in with the stool or mucous.

- It worried you as you looked this up online and it mentioned this may be a sign of cancer. You are now convinced you may have cancer.

- You hope today that the doctor can reassure you about these symptoms.

- You have not had any change in your bowel habits.

- If asked, you do admit to having quite firm stools, particularly when you are at work and you don't drink much fluid in the day.

- If asked, you often have to strain when going to the toilet to open your bowels.

- You have not lost any weight.

- You have no abdominal pain.

- There is no family history of bowel cancer.

- If the doctor asks to examine you today, you agree to abdominal examination but decline rectal examination.

- If the doctor explains, without using jargon, that this sounds like an anal fissure, you accept the explanation. You agree to try measures at home to soften your stool, including increasing your fluid intake. You are not keen on taking a laxative at this stage.

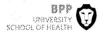

Data gathering, technical and assessment skills

History

- It is important to firstly establish what the three issues are so that you can manage the consultation effectively.

- Once you have established what these problems are, then carry out your data gathering for them, bearing in mind it is likely you will only be able to cover one issue.

If discussing the foot pain:

- How long has she had the pain? Was the onset gradual or sudden?

- Any history of trauma or injury?

- Any clear trigger that she can identify?

- Does she notice that anything makes the pain worse? Does movement or rest make it worse?

- Has she tried anything to try to settle it? What has worked? What hasn't?

- Are there any associated symptoms? Redness? Heat? Swelling?

If discussing the 'stye':

- What does she mean by a stye? What symptoms did she have exactly?

- Where was this lump?

- Did it cause her any irritation/pain?

- Did it cause any visual disturbance? Red eye?

- How long did it last? How did it resolve? What did she do to help it resolve?

If discussing the rectal bleeding:

- How long has this been going on for? On how many occasions?

- How much blood is there?

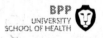

- What is the colour of the blood? Is it fresh red or is it dark?

- Is it mixed in with the stool or is it separate?

- Did any pain accompany the passing of blood?

- What are her bowels like usually? Is she constipated? Has she had any change in her bowel habits?

- Any weight loss? Abdominal pain? Loss of appetite?

- Has she ever had this before? If so, was she given any treatment?

- Any family history of bowel problems – ask about bowel cancer specifically.

Red flags
Rectal bleeding (under the age of 50)
- Weight loss
- Persistent unexplained abdominal pain
- Rectal or abdominal mass on examination
- Iron deficiency anaemia
- Altered bowel habits

Examination
- Abdominal examination and offer rectal examination (with chaperone)

Findings:

- Abdominal examination normal – soft, non-tender, no masses or herniae

- Rectal examination – declined by patient today

Interpersonal skills

Ideas, concerns, expectations

- Managing a list is something that most candidates dread! It is something that isn't often covered in courses or books, possibly because it can be difficult to use a consultation structure when managing these patients.

- However, it is useful to practise this, not only for CSA but also for clinical practice.

- Here are a few tips:

  - Watch your body language when a patient presents with a list – many people will subconsciously sink back into the chair, or look slightly irritated – make sure you remain engaged and interested!

  - Start the consultation by recognising there is more than one issue – 'I can see there are a few things concerning you today.'

  - Establish which are most concerning to the patient. There may be a discrepancy between which is the most concerning to the patient and which is clinically the most urgent – eg 'I can see that you are worried about your ingrowing toenail, but I am a little concerned about your vaginal bleeding, would it be ok to start with this?'

  - Prioritise tasks sensitively; the patient may feel that you are dismissing them if you do not address that these issues are concerning to them – 'These are all important problems, and I want to make sure we give each the time they deserve. To ensure that we can do this properly we may need to bring you back for another appointment, how does this sound to you?'

  - This approach is far more likely to enable you to move forwards with the consultation than an approach of 'One appointment means one problem' which the patient may find antagonistic in the CSA.

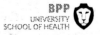
BPP
UNIVERSITY
SCHOOL OF HEALTH

It is still possible to keep to a structure:

- Establish their reason for attending today – What is worrying her and which does she think is most important?

- Identify that there are multiple issues and work with the patient to prioritise the tasks (this can demonstrate shared management).

- Prioritise one of the problems to discuss today – negotiating with the patient what you feel is the most clinically important and which they feel is concerning them the most, and use whatever consultation model to discuss this one problem.

- Safety net for this problem.

- Arrange to follow up, or signpost to appropriate services (eg optician/physiotherapist) to discuss the other issues to show that you have not dismissed them.

Clinical management

- The main focus of management will be addressing that you will need to prioritise tasks and identify which is potentially the concerning issue that needs to be dealt with first.

- In this case, the rectal bleeding is potentially a serious problem and so this should be your priority to discuss first.

- If you addressed the stye and foot pain first, you will not have time to discuss the rectal bleeding and could miss something serious, so you will need to identify the red flag symptom when a patient presents with a list.

- The history and examination suggests this lady has an anal fissure. She has painful rectal bleeding with a history of straining and constipation.

- Ideally, you would like to perform a rectal examination – you could invite her to return for this if she declines examination today.

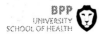

- Explain to her that an anal fissure is a small tear in the lining of the rectum, which usually occurs from straining and passing very firm stool.

- You could explain that this can lead to a cycle of avoiding passing stool due to fear of pain, which can worsen the constipation and exacerbate symptoms.

- You need to aim to break this cycle by avoiding constipation – you can try to tackle this with diet and lifestyle measures – she mentioned that when she doesn't drink enough fluid she has firmer stool, so she may want to just aim to increase fluid intake, or you could discuss stool softeners. This is an opportunity to discuss changes she can make, and interventions you can offer, demonstrating shared care management.

- It is also important to educate this lady that she should avoid straining, which can exacerbate symptoms.

- You could also discuss topical therapies – you could suggest that if symptoms persist you could offer her topical anaesthetic, or topical GTN ointment (which will act by relaxing the anal sphincter). As she had symptoms for two days and things have settled, this isn't necessary at this stage, but you could discuss that these options are available if symptoms recur.

- Invite her to return to discuss her stye and foot pain in more detail if time doesn't allow in this consultation.

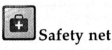
Safety net

- Advise her to return if she experiences any further rectal bleeding, particularly as she hasn't been examined on this occasion.

- Invite her to return for rectal examination.

- Advise her of red flags and to return if present: weight loss, abdominal pain, change in bowel habit, or recurrent rectal bleeding.

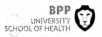

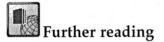
Further reading

1. NICE CKS (2016) *Anal Fissure*. [Online]. Available at:
   https://cks.nice.org.uk/anal-fissure
   [Accessed 11 February 2017].

2. GP Notebook (2017) *Anal fissure*.
   http://gpnotebook.co.uk/simplepage.cfm?ID=-66715648
   [Accessed 28 February 2017].

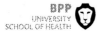

37. Rheumatoid arthritis

Instructions to candidates

Name:	Belinda Beech
Age:	53 years old
Past medical history:	Post-natal depression
	Eczema
Occupation:	Cleaner
Social history:	Smoker 10 cigarettes/day
	Alcohol 4 units/week

Instructions to patients

Opening statement

> *I think I've got arthritis.*

Background

- You are Belinda, a 53-year-old cleaner.

- Over the last eight weeks you have been struggling with pains in your hands.

- It is causing you a lot of pain in the morning and you have requested a later start at work. Your employer hasn't been very understanding, because by the time they get into work your pain has improved.

- You have noticed your knuckles are painful and swollen, particularly in the morning.

- You have also had pains in some of your fingers – if asked specifically, you point to all your knuckles and the small joints on your first and second fingers and your thumbs.

BPP
UNIVERSITY
SCHOOL OF HEALTH

- If asked, you are well in yourself. You state that you are always quite tired, but you have always attributed this to your busy lifestyle.

- If asked, you have not had any weight loss, sweats or fevers.

- You have tried paracetamol but it hasn't helped very much.

- You work full time as a cleaner at a shopping centre.

- You live with your 2 children (aged 16 and 18 years old) and your partner.

- There is no history of any trauma or injury.

- If asked, you think this may be arthritis as your grandmother had arthritis and she ended up with permanent deformities of her hand. You are worried this might happen to you.

- You are hoping that the doctor will agree to write a note to your employer supporting your case for a later start at work.

- Your expectation today is to leave with some stronger analgesia.

- If the doctor suggests you need to see a specialist, you are quite surprised, but agree to the appointment, as you would like this to be resolved promptly.

Data gathering, technical and assessment skills

History

- Establish exactly what has been going on – why does she think she has arthritis?

- What symptoms is she getting?

- Where is she getting the joint pains? Which joints specifically?

- Is it unilateral or bilateral?

- Are any other joints affected?

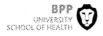

- Does she notice any pattern to the pain? Be specific – is it worse in the morning or the evening? Is it worse on movement or at rest?

- Is there any associated stiffness/swelling/redness/warmth?

- Is she systemically well (fever, weight loss)?

- How long has this been going on for? Is it getting better/worse/staying the same?

- What has she tried for this already? Any painkillers? Did they help?

- She mentioned her grandmother had arthritis – does she know what sort of arthritis this was?

- Any significant medical history? It may be useful to ask specifically about relevant conditions eg psoriasis.

- Any regular medication or allergies? – this can be useful when deciding on drug management.

Examination
- A structured examination of the hands: look, feel, move and functionality.

- Look at which joints are affected – DIPJ/ PIPJ/ MCPJs?

- Are they red or swollen?

- Are there any obvious deformities? – Z-thumb, Boutonnière, swan neck deformity.

- Any rheumatoid nodules? Any Heberdens or Bouchards nodes to suggest osteoarthritis?

- Feel the joints – do they feel warm? Are they boggy? Squeeze the MCPJs – if tender this may suggest rheumatoid arthritis.

- Move – ask the patient to make a fist, and then stretch out her hands. Ask them to put their hands into a prayer sign and a reverse prayer.

- Functionality – assess their ability to pick up a button, hold a pen and do up a button.

Findings in this case:

- Red, slightly warm MCPJs symmetrically on both hands. Tender to squeeze and feel boggy. Boggy swelling of PIPs (proximal interphalangeal joints) on first and second fingers bilaterally.

- Pain and stiffness on making a fist. Other movements not affected.

- Swelling of PIPJs leading to early appearances of Boutonnière deformity of first finger left hand.

Interpersonal skills

- It is important to learn what impact this is having on her at home and at work. This is the prompt in her consulting today; try to explore the psychosocial aspects of this:

  - Have you discussed this with your boss? What changes do you think need to be made? Are there any ways you think we can help you with this? Eg fit note with amended duties or altered hours, occupational health assessment.

  - Is this impacting on any activities that you like to do outside of work? Occupational therapy and physiotherapy may be useful sources to signpost patients towards. In time, orthotics or medical appliances may also need to become involved if deformity ensues.

Ideas, concerns, expectations

- She mentioned that she thought this was arthritis; what drew her to this conclusion? Was there anything else she thought this could be?

- Was there anything in particular that worried her if it was arthritis?

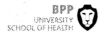

- If she has mentioned about her grandmother, echo this back to show you are actively listening – you said that your grandmother had some deformity to her hands, is this why you were worried about your hand pains?

- Try to learn what she was hoping to get from today's consultation – 'Sometimes people have ideas about how best to investigate or manage this, did you have any thoughts about this?'

Clinical management

- This is a case of a new diagnosis of an inflammatory arthritis – in this case rheumatoid arthritis is most likely.

- Check her understanding of this diagnosis then explain it without using jargon.

- Explain that diagnosis is usually a clinical diagnosis, but can be supported by blood tests, which may show raised inflammatory markers, positive rheumatoid factor and changes on x-rays.

- You could therefore arrange blood tests and an x-ray (important to explain to the patient what you are checking on the blood tests and why – 'I would like to check a blood test to measure the level of inflammation in your blood, and also measure something called rheumatoid factor, which can be raised.'). You may also want to check ANA and anti-CCP antibodies which may also be raised.

- It is important to mention that rheumatoid factor can be negative even in cases of rheumatoid arthritis, but if it is positive it makes the diagnosis more likely.

- However, do not delay referral to await results of the blood tests and x-rays if you clinically suspect rheumatoid arthritis. If this is the case, seek consent to make an urgent referral to a rheumatologist.

- Urgent referral is indicated if small joints are affected, more than one joint is affected or there is a delay in symptom onset and presentation of more than three months[1].

- You could also discuss with her that early assessment is needed to try to prevent deformity.

- You may want to discuss with her possible treatments – disease modifying anti-rheumatic drugs (DMARDs), which require regular monitoring.

- In the meantime, make a plan with the patient about how you will manage her symptoms:

  - Does she need a note to her employer so she can have adaptations of altered duties at work?

  - Would she like any additional analgesia? – discuss starting an NSAID which may help her symptomatically.

  - You could discuss with her about occupational therapy adaptations if this is necessary.

Safety net

- This may be quite overwhelming and a lot of information. It may be useful to offer her some written information on rheumatoid arthritis – useful information on Arthritis Research UK website also. This website offers useful information on self-help measures as well eg exercises that might be beneficial.

- Offer to review her once she has seen the rheumatologist and to help monitor her response to treatment.

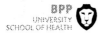

Further reading

1. NICE (2015) *Rheumatoid arthritis in adults: management.* [Online]. Available at: www.nice.org.uk/guidance/CG79 [Accessed 11 February 2017].

2. SIGN (2011) *Management of early rheumatoid arthritis.* [Online]. Available at: www.sign.ac.uk/pdf/sign123.pdf [Accessed 11 February 2017].

3. Arthritis Research Council (2017) *Rheumatoid Arthritis.* [Online]. Available at: www.arthritisresearchuk.org/arthritis -information/conditions/rheumatoid-arthritis.aspx [Accessed 28 February 2017].

38. Stress incontinence

Instructions to candidates

Name:	Amelia Morton
Age:	40 years old
Past medical history:	Nil
Occupation:	Housewife
Social history:	Never smoked
	No alcohol

Instructions to patients

Opening statement

I need some help with my waterworks, doctor.

Background

- You are Amelia, a 49-year-old housewife.

- You have noticed over the last year that you are leaking urine.

- If asked, you state that it seems to be worse when you are laughing or running. You have recently started going to the gym to try to lose weight and when you are running you have to wear sanitary pads. You are finding this frustrating.

- If asked, you are able to control your bladder when you get the urge to go to the toilet.

- You have not increased your frequency of going to the toilet to empty your bladder.

- You have no night-time symptoms.

- If asked, you have no pain/burning on urination and you have not seen any blood in your urine.

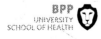

38. Stress incontinence

- You do not take any regular medication.

- You have no significant medical history.

- You have never smoked and are a life-long teetotaller.

- There is no history of abdominal surgery.

- You are otherwise well in yourself, with no other medical conditions.

- If asked, you have 3 children aged 16, 12 and 9 years old. If asked, you had a forceps delivery on your first delivery and normal vaginal delivery with your second and third children.

- If asked, you don't recall being told your children were particularly big when born – they were all around 7 lb (3 kg).

- If asked, you haven't noticed any pain during sexual intercourse or dryness of your vagina. You are still having periods and they are regular.

- If asked, you do admit to being slightly constipated from time to time. This is how you have always been and there is no change in your bowel habits.

- The main impact this is having on you is your ability to go to the gym, which you were starting to enjoy.

- If asked, you are hoping to be prescribed some medication to help with your symptoms.

- If, however, the doctor explains clearly the diagnosis of stress incontinence and the causes of this, you would be willing to accept referral for supervised pelvic floor exercises.

- If the doctor discusses surgical options with you, this isn't something you would want to consider at the moment.

Data gathering, technical and assessment skills

History

- What symptoms is she having?

- How long has this been going on for?

- Is there any particular pattern to the urine leakage? Are there any particular circumstances where she notices these symptoms? Does anything make them worse?

- Determine what type of incontinence she has:

  - Stress – does she get leakage when coughing/straining/laughing/exertion?

  - Urge/Overactive bladder – does she have to frequently go to the toilet? Does she pass a good amount of urine or is it frequent small amounts? Once she's been to the toilet does her bladder feel empty? Is she able to hold her bladder when she feels the urge to urinate? How long can she hold her bladder for? Does she get any night-time symptoms?

- Rule out other causes:

  - Haematuria? – consider bladder carcinoma
  - Dysuria? – consider UTI
  - Polydipsia? – consider diabetes

- Ask about risk factors:

  - Obstetric history – how many pregnancies? Vaginal delivery? Macrosomia? Instrumental delivery?

  - Constipation – straining may weaken pelvic floor

  - Chronic cough

  - Obesity

  - Caffeine and carbonated drinks (for urge incontinence)

  - Abdominal or pelvic surgery

  - Prolapse

  - Urogenital atrophy – ask about vaginal dryness, dyspareunia

213

Red flags
- Pelvic mass
- Haematuria – suggestive of bladder cancer

Examination
- Abdominal examination – looking for a palpable bladder (suggesting chronic retention leading to overflow incontinence), or any abdominal masses (that might be increasing intra-abdominal pressure).

- Pelvic examination – assess for prolapse, leakage on coughing and feel the strength of pelvic floor muscle contractions.

  This will obviously not be expected to be done in the exam, but ask to do it, as you would in a normal consultation, and explain what you will be examining for and why – it is important that you explain to the patient why you are doing a certain examination so that you can seek informed consent.

- Urine dipstick in all patients – looking for signs of urine infection or haematuria.

- It might also be useful to check BMI.

Examination findings:

- Abdominal examination normal
- Pelvic examination declined
- BMI 29
- Urine dip normal

Interpersonal skills

Ideas, concerns, expectations

- Enquire about how this is affecting her life – is it stopping her from doing things she would normally like to do?

- She mentioned it is occurring when she is running – how does this make her feel? What impact has this had?

- Find out what she thought is going on. What does she think is causing this?

214

- What is concerning her about it? She says it has been going on for a year, so has something changed or worried her to cause her to consult about it now?

- Has she tried anything already to manage this? How does she feel this could be managed, or how was she hoping you may be able to help with this?

Clinical management

- This is a case of stress urinary incontinence – explain this diagnosis to the patient without using jargon.

  - Eg the bladder is surrounded by muscles that support it from beneath. This prevents you from leaking urine. If these muscles become weakened, they aren't able to prevent your bladder from leaking when the pressure in your tummy rises through things like coughing, laughing or running.

- Explain risk factors:

  - Eg this is caused, or can be made worse by factors that increase the pressure in your abdomen – eg constipation, obesity, chronic cough and/or factors that weaken your pelvic floor, such as childbirth.

- Offer referral for supervised pelvic floor training – this is often available through local incontinence or physiotherapy services.

- Whilst awaiting referral to bladder training services you could advise her on pelvic floor exercises – there are some useful leaflets that can explain how to do this (see 'Further reading' for a link to one from www.nhs.uk).

- After explaining the risk factors you can discuss how you can manage these – this lady mentioned she is prone to constipation, so you could try managing this also:

  - This can be managed with lifestyle changes initially – increasing fibre and fluid intake.

- If this doesn't improve things you could consider starting laxatives.

- Encourage her to continue exercising; she has taken a positive step here to try to lose weight, which will help with these symptoms as well as having benefits on heart health, mood etc.

- You can discuss with her that if pelvic floor exercises are unsuccessful the next step would be referral to a urogynaecologist to consider surgical options:

  - Patients may want to enquire about what the surgical options are; it may be useful to know a bit more about what these are. They include colposuspension (a procedure that lifts up the bladder neck) and trans-vaginal tape (a procedure that provides support and lifts the urethra).

  - If they are not keen to consider surgical options, you could consider prescribing duloxetine.

Safety net

- Offer to review her following her supervised pelvic floor muscle training to monitor progress.

- Advise her to see a doctor if she experiences haematuria.

Further reading

1. NICE CKS (2015) *Incontinence – urinary, in women*. [Online]. Available at: https://cks.nice.org.uk/incontinence-urinary -in-women [Accessed 12 February 2017]

2. NHS UK (2008) *Pelvic floor exercises – for women*. [Online]. Available at: www.nhs.uk/Planners/pregnancycareplanner/ Documents/BandBF_pelvic_floor_women.pdf [Accessed 12 February 2017].

39. Chronic kidney disease

Instructions to candidates

Name:	Graham Elder
Age:	75 years old
Past medical history:	Hypertension
Medication:	Amlodipine 5 mg od
Social history:	Never smoked
	No alcohol

Blood results:

	2 weeks ago	3 months ago	4 months ago	
Hb	14.5	14.2	14.5	(13 – 18 g/dL)
MCV	82	80	81	(80 – 100 fL)
MCH	31	33	33	(27 – 33 pg)
Platelets	186	194	191	(150 – 400 × 10^9/L)
WCC	5.4	5.7	5.5	(4 – 11 × 10^9/L)
Urea	6.2	6.7	6.6	(3 – 6.5 mmol/L)
Creatinine	105	110	102	(60 – 125 µmol/L)
Na	138	137	138	(135 – 145 mmol/L)
K	4.2	4.4	4.4	(3.5 – 5 mmol/L)
GFR	47	51	46	(> 60 ml/min)
ACR	1.5	-	-	(< 3 mg/mmol)

At last review:
Brief discussion about likely diagnosis of CKD and need for repeat blood test to confirm. Discussed BP, not well controlled (156/92 today).

Plan:
Repeat blood tests with urine ACR in six months and review. Repeat BP at review.

Instructions to patients

Opening statement

> *You called me in to discuss my blood tests doctor.*

Background

- You are Graham, a 75-year-old retired solicitor.

- You were called in to discuss your results, which were done as a follow-up from your previous consultation.

- You were told at your last review that there was a problem with your kidneys and you wonder if your kidneys are now failing.

- You feel well in yourself – you have no weight loss/fatigue or systemic upset.

- You deny any urinary symptoms – you have no discomfort on urination, frequency or urgency of urination and no history of blood in your urine.

- If asked, you have no previous medical conditions apart from 'a bit of blood pressure'.

- If asked, you have not taken any non-prescribed medication recently.

- You take your amlodipine regularly – once daily for your blood pressure.

- If asked, you have never smoked and do not drink any alcohol.

- You live with your wife. You mobilise independently.

- You are quite concerned that you were called in for your blood results today. You have been speaking to your daughter, who is a nurse, and you discussed that if there was a problem with your kidneys you would like a referral to see a kidney specialist.

- You are quite concerned as you have been reading about kidney disease and worried that you may end up needing dialysis.

- This concerns you as your neighbour goes for dialysis and has to miss going bowling. You also enjoy going bowling and wouldn't want to give this up.

- If the doctor gives a clear explanation of why you don't need a referral to a kidney specialist, you will accept this and get 'on board' with medical management.

- If the doctor then discusses medication, you are wary of adding too many medications at one time, so would like to just add one today if this is needed. You would be happy to add in other medication later, if this is necessary.

- If, however, they dismiss your concerns you will demand to see a kidney specialist and refuse to move on from this point.

Data gathering, technical and assessment skills

History

- Find out more about why he had the blood tests – were they routine or was he having symptoms?

- This patient has CKD – enquire about risk factors:
  - Any significant medical history – ask specifically about diabetes, hypertension, previous kidney problems, cardiac disease.
  - Any regular medication? Including over the counter medication (eg regular NSAID use).

- Does he smoke?

- Does he have any symptoms of CKD? – weakness/lethargy/ fatigue/oedema/SOB?

39. Chronic kidney disease

- Does he have any symptoms that may point to another cause – frank haematuria? Or any symptoms suggestive of a urinary tract infection – dysuria/frequency/urgency?

- It might also be useful to ask about his social circumstances – who does he live with? How does he mobilise?

Red flags
- Any signs or symptoms of urological cancer – eg haematuria

- Palpable bladder on examination – suggests urinary retention

---

Examination
- Check for any signs of fluid overload – oedema (ankle or sacral), pleural effusions on chest auscultation

- Examine for a palpable bladder on abdominal examination (chronic retention can lead to renal impairment)

- Check BP

Examination findings:

- BP 186/95
- Clinically euvolaemic
- Abdominal examination normal. No palpable bladder

Interpersonal skills

Ideas, concerns, expectations

- Did this patient have any thoughts on what his blood tests might show?

- Explore what he understands by the term CKD – is this something he has heard of before? What has been explained to him already? Does it make him think of anything in particular? Does anything worry him about this?

- Explore any concerns he has about this diagnosis and why he has these concerns.

- What are his thoughts about the management of this? Does he have any expectations of how this might be managed?

Clinical management

- This patient has CKD – explain this diagnosis without using jargon.

- Reassure him that this is common – statistics vary, but about 1/10 to 1/20 people will have a GFR < 60[1,2] and its prevalence increases with age.

- You can reassure him that it often causes no symptoms and is usually picked up incidentally on routine blood tests.

- You could also explain risk factors for CKD – hypertension, diabetes etc making this relevant to his case.

- After exploring this patient's concern that this may progress to dialysis it is important to reassure him that this is only for end stage renal failure, and he is not at that stage as his renal function is stable and only mildly reduced currently.

- You could explain that by managing his risk factors you can try to slow the rate of progression, and this may help him comply with management, given his concerns about progression to dialysis.

- Optimisation of blood pressure is likely to be your main priority here.

  - His urinary ACR is normal.

  - The next line of management would be an angiotensin converting enzyme inhibitor (ACEi) or angiotensin II receptor blocker (ARB). You could explain to him that this will help protect his kidneys.

  - Aim for BP < 140/90.

- When starting an ACEi it is important to inform him that you will need to re-check his renal function within two weeks to check that it hasn't deteriorated.

- Discuss with him managing risk factors:

  - CKD is associated with cardiovascular disease, so you will need to discuss managing cardiovascular risk factors. You could discuss starting atorvastatin 20 mg as primary prevention.

  - For this reason, you could also discuss starting low dose aspirin.

  - If you don't have time to discuss this, at least mention that there are other factors to discuss, to show the examiner you are aware of this and can prioritise tasks.

- Discuss the monitoring that is involved – he will need annual blood test and urinary ACR.

- At this stage of renal impairment, he will need to have his renal function monitored yearly, but if he is showing rapid signs of progression, he would need more frequent monitoring.

- You could offer him a written information leaflet on CKD; patient.co.uk offers a useful leaflet, that will outline this information and management; again, with all leaflets it is important to explain what information there is on the leaflet.

Safety net

  - As you are likely to be starting an ACEi today you will need to recheck his renal function within two weeks and review BP following this.

  - You will need to then monitor renal function on an annual basis currently.

  - Advise him that if he has any intercurrent illnesses, for example D&V, he is at risk of acute or chronic kidney injury as a result of dehydration. Therefore it is important to seek a review early and maintain hydration.

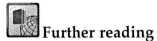

Further reading

1. Aitken GR et al. Change in prevalence of chronic kidney disease in England over time: comparison of nationally representative cross-sectional surveys from 2003-2010. *BMJ Open* 2014; 4:e005480. http://bmjopen.bmj.com/content/4/9/e005480.full [Accessed 12 February 2017].

2. SIGN (2015) *Diagnosis and Management of Chronic Kidney Disease*. [Online]. Available at: www.sign.ac.uk/guidelines/fulltext/103/ [Accessed 12 February 2017].

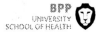

39. Chronic kidney disease

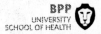

Index

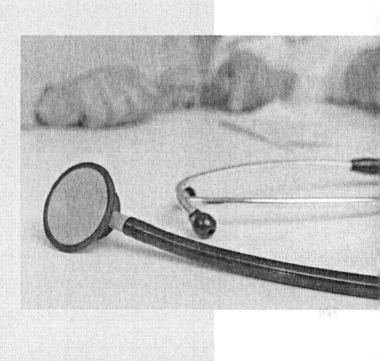

Index

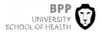

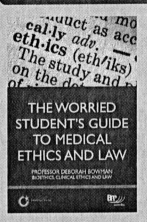

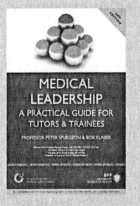

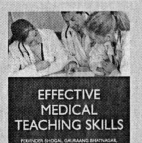

More titles in the Progressing your Medical Career Series

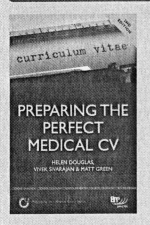

Are you unsure of how to structure your Medical CV? Would you like to know how to ensure you stand out from the crowd?

With competition for medical posts at an all time high it is vital that your Medical CV stands out over your fellow applicants. This comprehensive, unique and easy-to-read guide has been written with this in mind to help prospective medical students, current medical students and doctors of all grades prepare a Medical CV of the highest quality. Whether you are applying to medical school, currently completing your medical degree or a doctor progressing through your career (foundation doctor, specialty trainee in general practice, surgery or medicine, GP career grade or Consultant) this guide includes specific guidance for applicants at every level.

This time-saving and detailed guide:

- Explains what selection panels are looking for when reviewing applications at all levels

- Discusses how to structure your Medical CV to ensure you stand out for the right reasons

- Explores what information to include (and not to include) in your CV

- Covers what to consider when maintaining a portfolio at every step of your career, including, for revalidation and relicensing purposes

- Provides examples of high quality CVs to illustrate the above

This unique guide will show you how to prepare your CV for every step of your medical career from pre-Medical School right through to Consultant level and should be a constant companion to ensure you secure your first choice post every time.

£19.99
October 2011
Paperback
978-1-445381-62-6

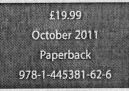

BPP
UNIVERSITY
SCHOOL OF HEALTH

www.bpp.com/health

More titles in the Progressing your Medical Career Series

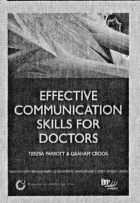

EFFECTIVE COMMUNICATION SKILLS FOR DOCTORS

TERESA PARROTT & GRAHAM CROOK

£19.99
September 2011
Paperback
978-1-445379-56-2

Would you like to know how to improve your communication skills? Are you looking for a clearly written book which explores all aspects of effective medical communication?

There is an urgent need to improve doctors' communication skills. Research has shown that poor communication can contribute to patient dissatisfaction, lack of compliance and increased medico-legal problems. Improved communication skills will impact positively on all of these areas. The last fifteen years have seen unprecedented changes in medicine and the role of doctors. Effective communication skills are vital to these new roles. But communication is not just related to personality. Skills can be learned which can make your communication more effective, and help you to improve your relationships with patients, their families and fellow doctors.

This book shows how to learn those skills and outlines why we all need to communicate more effectively. Healthcare is increasingly a partnership. Change is happening at all levels, from government directives to patient expectations. Communication is a bridge between the wisdom of the past and the vision of the future.

Readers of this book can also gain free access to an online module which upon successful completion can download a certificate for their portfolio of learning/ Revalidation/CPD records.

This easy-to-read guide will help medical students and doctors at all stages of their careers improve their communication within a hospital environment.

BPP
UNIVERSITY
SCHOOL OF HEALTH

www.bpp.com/health

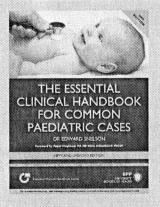
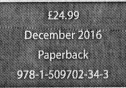

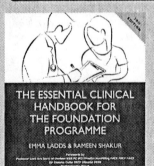